490

THE HISTORY OF AMERICAN EPIDEMIOLOGY

THE HISTORY OF
AMERICAN EPIDEMIOLOGY

BY

C.-E. A. WINSLOW, Dr.P.H.

Professor Emeritus, Yale University School of Medicine;
Editor, American Journal of Public Health

WILSON G. SMILLIE, M.D.

Professor and Chairman, Department of Public Health and
Preventive Medicine, Cornell University Medical College

JAMES A. DOULL, M.D.

Medical Director, Leonard Wood Memorial
(American Leprosy Foundation)

JOHN E. GORDON, M.D.

Professor and Chairman, Department of Epidemiology,
School of Public Health, Harvard University

Edited by

FRANKLIN H. TOP, M.D.

Professor of Epidemiology and Pediatrics, College of
Medical Sciences, University of Minnesota

Sponsored by
The Epidemiology Section,
American Public Health Association

ST. LOUIS
THE C. V. MOSBY COMPANY
1952

Printed in the
United States of America

Press of
The C. V. Mosby Company
St. Louis

FOREWORD

The four chapters in this monograph were presented in part at the Twentieth Anniversary Session of the Epidemiology Section of the American Public Health Association held in New York City, October 27, 1949. Attendance at the meeting was large, and a canvass midway in the program gave evidence of a great interest and resulted in a virtual mandate by the audience to preserve in more tangible form the contributions being presented at the anniversary session. As a consequence, publication of the four papers, subsequently augmented, was decided upon after consultation with the authors and with the Executive Secretary of the American Public Health Association. This monograph, then, is sponsored by the Epidemiology Section of the American Public Health Association with the consent of the parent organization.

The editorial tasks involved were not burdensome but the absorption in other affairs on the part of the authors delayed somewhat the present appearance of the contributions in book form. The historical record is as timely, however, in 1952. Few changes were felt necessary or desirable and no attempt was made to reduce the length, to follow a set pattern, or to alter style. There is some repetition in historical background material in the sections subsequent to the first, but this fact lends considerably to setting the stage for the recital of events of the particular era being discussed and for interpretation of these events.

One might question the desirability of marking a twentieth anniversary when the more commonly commemorated quarter century is so close. The founding of the Epidemiology Section of the American Public Health Association in 1929 is a fairly recent event when measured by other Sections in the same organization and by similar scientific groups elsewhere. Nevertheless, it beckoned as a noteworthy milestone. We had discussed the desirability of presenting before the Epidemiology Section the historical studies of Professor Winslow on Colonial Epidemiology and those of Professor Smillie on the Era of Great Epidemics. What could be more appropriate than commemorating an anniversary with such interesting researches, and why not complete the historical picture and devote an entire session to a symposium on the topic,

5

"The History of American Epidemiology"? Submission of the idea to Officers and Council Members of the Section met with wholehearted approval. Happily, Professor Doull agreed to discuss the Bacteriological Era and Professor Gordon the period from 1920 to the present; both are eminently capable by experience and bent to cover the respective periods assigned.

The title and the content of this monograph may appear at first glance and reading to be rather provincial. Science is universal and as Goethe has stated, "Art and science . . . belong to the world at large and before them vanish all limits of nationality." American contributions to epidemiology must of necessity be considered as fairly recent additions to the sum total of knowledge in this field. The infectious diseases that scourged the American continent were brought by settlers and tradesmen from the four corners of the world, and knowledge concerning them and their control was largely the result of Old World thought and indoctrination; certainly this was true in colonial times. It is noteworthy that each of the contributors to this volume documents and credits Old World ideas and thought and emphasizes their influence upon happenings in the New World. Granting the premise, it appeared desirable to record, at least in part, contributions to epidemiology made by American workers.

Needless to say, the authors of this monograph have brought to their task knowledge, insight, and scholarly treatment. This volume should become a cherished document of American contributions to epidemiology by all persons interested in medical and public health matters.

FRANKLIN H. TOP, M.D.

Secretary, Epidemiology Section,
American Public Health Association, 1949

Officers of Section, 1949:

John J. Phair, M.D., Chairman
Hollis C. Ingraham, M.D., Vice Chairman
Franklin H. Top, M.D., Secretary

CONTENTS

PAGE

FOREWORD _ _ _ _ _ _ _ _ _ _ _ _ _ _ 5

FRANKLIN H. TOP

I

THE COLONIAL ERA AND THE FIRST YEARS OF
THE REPUBLIC (1607-1799) THE PESTILENCE
THAT WALKETH IN DARKNESS _ _ _ _ _ 11

C.-E. A. WINSLOW

II

THE PERIOD OF GREAT EPIDEMICS IN THE
UNITED STATES (1800-1875) _ _ _ _ _ _ 52

WILSON G. SMILLIE

III

THE BACTERIOLOGICAL ERA (1876-1920) _ _ _ _ 74

JAMES A. DOULL

IV

THE TWENTIETH CENTURY—YESTERDAY, TO-
DAY, AND TOMORROW (1920-_ _ _ _) _ _ _ _ 114

JOHN E. GORDON

THE HISTORY OF AMERICAN EPIDEMIOLOGY

THE HISTORY OF
AMERICAN EPIDEMIOLOGY

I. THE COLONIAL ERA AND THE FIRST YEARS
OF THE REPUBLIC (1607-1799)—THE PESTILENCE
THAT WALKETH IN DARKNESS

C.-E. A. WINSLOW, DR. P.H., F.A.P.H.A.*

FOR the first century and a half of colonial life, there was no "epidemiology" in America; but there was an abundance of epidemics.

The account by George Percy of the settlement at Jamestown,[7] after recounting a series of deaths, says, "Our men were destroyed with cruell diseases, as Swellings, Fluxes, Burning Fevers, and by warres, and some departed suddenly, but for the most part they died of meere famine. There were never Englishmen left in a forreigne countrey in such miserie as wee were in this new discovered Virginia."

Shattuck[16] states that three months after the arrival of the Pilgrims at Plymouth fifty-five only survived, out of an original company of one hundred and one. "The sick were destitute of almost all the comforts which their miserable condition rendered indispensable. Their sufferings were increased by the want of well persons to perform the duties among the sick; there being, at one time, not more than six or seven persons in tolerable health."

The first recorded epidemic on this continent actually occurred in New England two years before the Plymouth landing.[16, 19] Captain Dermer, an English adventurer, passed the winter of 1618-1619 in a New England harbor and observed it. Its effects were still obvious when the Pilgrims arrived. The Indian warriors were "reduced from nine thousand to a few hundreds." The Massachusetts tribe alone was supposed to have lost 2,700 out of 3,000 persons. Dermer described this disease as the "plague"; Hutchinson thought it was smallpox. Gookin quotes Indian survivors who reported that,

---

*Editor American Journal of Public Health. Contribution from the Historical Library, Yale School of Medicine.

11

among the victims, "the bodies all over were exceeding yellow (describing it by a yellow garment they showed me), both before they died and afterwards." Webster[19] was therefore convinced that this was yellow fever, which seems highly improbable since it occurred in the winter season.

Throughout the Seventeenth and early Eighteenth Centuries we find numerous records of devastating epidemics. In 1631, "the smallpox, first breaking out at Saugus, spread from Narragansett to Piscataqua, and westward to the Connecticut River and swept off entire villages of the Indians. Two years later, a similar epidemic occurred and "made great devastations among the unfortunate native races of Massachusetts." In 1638, 1644, 1646, 1647, and 1649, there were records of fasts held for deliverance from unusual sickness, and thanksgiving services after such deliverance —all in the Massachusetts Colony or towns within that Colony.

In 1647, there was a malignant fever in the summer and an epidemic influenza (of low virulence) in the winter, in New England. A similar outbreak of respiratory disease occurred in 1655; and, in 1659, in the same area, the first recorded epidemic of diphtheria appeared.

Between 1665 and 1675, smallpox was epidemic in Europe and in 1677 and 1678 in New England. In 1668, there was an outbreak of yellow fever in New York.

In the winter of 1697-1698, all New England suffered from a very severe epidemic of influenza. "Whole families and whole towns were seized nearly at the same time." In 1702, and again in 1721, Boston had severe epidemics of smallpox. In the latter year, more than one-half the inhabitants (5,759) of the city had the disease and 844 died. Aside from such major epidemics as those mentioned, early colonial records are, of course, full of references to "bilious fevers," "agues," and the like, particularly in outlying settlements. These were, no doubt, in large measure, typhoid fever, dysenteries, and malaria. The difficulties in diagnosing outbreaks from such records are, however, illustrated in one epidemic of the "burning ague" which occurred in various parts of Rhode Island in 1723. "It did not prevail in a large town, but in villages, and perhaps the clearing of some neighboring swamps might have been one cause of the disease." Aha, you say, malaria. But "in proportion to its patients, no disease in America was ever so mortal."[19] Which leaves us wholly at a loss.

THE EPIDEMIC OF 1735-1740

In the year 1735, there occurred one of the most devastating of these early epidemics; and the only one which has been analyzed with really significant results. The study of this outbreak by Ernest Caulfield[4] is a masterpiece of intelligent epidemiology, conducted 200 years after the event. By an exhaustive study of town records and of gravestones of the period, Caulfield has established the following facts.

The primary outbreak began in May, 1735, in Kingston, N. H., where the "Throat Distemper" killed so many children (26 in the month of August alone) that the total number of deaths for the little town was 102 for the year, against a previous yearly average of less than 10. During the year, this same dreadful disease spread to the northeast, affecting village after village along the coast of New Hampshire and Maine. Between July, 1735, and July, 1736, fifteen New Hampshire communities experienced 954 deaths, of which 802 were of children under 10 years of age and 139 between 10 and 20 years.

The same disease spread to certain Massachusetts towns near the New Hampshire border. In Haverhill, with a population of about 1,200 people (fifteen miles from Kingston), the epidemic began in November, 1735. There were 116 deaths recorded in 1736 and 130 deaths in 1737, 98 per cent in children and youths under 20 years of age. The previous records of the town showed about 10 deaths a year, so that the "throat distemper" caused a mortality of about 9 per 1,000 population. It was said that "more than half of the Haverhill children died. At least sixty families lost two or more children; some of them lost four or five apiece. Twenty-three families were left childless."[4]

Now comes an intriguing complication. In the fall of 1735, when the New Hampshire epidemic had crossed the Merrimack River, the city of Boston became seriously disturbed. The selectmen invited the leading physicians to a conference, and, after mature deliberation, these physicians reported that the "Eastern Distemper" "was communicated by means of a bad Air and not by Contagion," a conclusion in the solid tradition of Sydenham. At the very moment, however, a young man named How was on his way from Exeter to Boston. He developed a sore throat and was treated by Zabdiel Boylston. When this became known, the selectmen wanted to quarantine How on an island in the harbor, but the fact that the doctors had declared the disease noncontagious blocked legal action. The patient died before this particular controversy was solved.

No new cases developed in the neighborhood where How had been domiciled; but before the end of the year, a "throat distemper" made itself clearly manifest in other areas of the city. A day of "Prayer and Humiliation with Fasting" was duly declared by the Governor, for January 8, 1736. The outbreak continued until the middle of 1736 and it was computed that one-fourth of the population had contracted the disease.

Out of some 4,000 cases, however, only 114 were fatal—a very different picture from the experience in New Hampshire. There was no doubt in the minds of the Boston physicians that the disease was the same as that which had prevailed in the Eastern Provinces. William Douglass published a detailed account of the epidemic, expounding this view and containing admirable clinical data. Dr. G. H. Weaver calls it "the first adequate clinical description of scarlet fever in English."

There were various theories to account for the difference in fatality in Boston and in the Eastern Provinces. Hugh Adams, pastor of the church at Durham attributed the low death rate in Massachusetts to the fact that the laws of that province demanded that ministers of the gospel should be promptly and adequately paid, which was not the case in New Hampshire. No wonder, he said, that an epidemic was raging in New Hampshire while Massachusetts was relatively free. On the other hand, the medical fraternity in Boston was quite convinced that the superiority of their treatment accounted for the difference. The Boston public were told on the front pages of their newspapers that the small-town physicians "altho' their bad Success evidently shews that they have no manner of Notion of the Nature of the Disease or Method of Cure yet persist in one invariable Method to kill very successfully, *secundem Artem.*"

Caulfield presents convincing evidence that both clergy and medical men were in error in their explanations. What happened was that New Hampshire and Maine and towns like Haverhill in Massachusetts suffered from a severe epidemic of diphtheria; while Boston had an epidemic of scarlet fever. The clinical symptoms which were clearly described in certain cases and the fatality rates of under 3 per cent in Boston and of 16-60 per cent in New Hampshire make this conclusion inescapable.

Finally, the situation was further complicated by an independent epidemic of diphtheria which began in New Jersey in 1735 and spread across to Connecticut in 1736. Both the northeastern and the southwestern outbreaks continued to extend toward each other but did not coalesce until 1740. In the five years 1735-1740, Caulfield estimates that some 2,000 deaths from the "throat distemper" occurred in New Hampshire and Maine in a population of 29,000, with an over-all mortality of about 14 per 1,000 population from this disease alone. In Massachusetts and Connecticut (where the disease was scarlet fever, not diphtheria), the excess mortality due to it was only 3 per 1,000.

THE WRATH OF GOD

Epidemiology must operate on a theory of causation; and, so far as the great mass of the population was concerned, there can be no doubt that prevailing theory attributed unusual epidemics of disease primarily to God's intent of punishing his children for their sins and recalling them to a better way of life. The Bible contains some thirty distinct references (all but two in the Old Testament) to pestilence as sent among the people by direct act of God.

Cotton Mather, one of the keenest minds of the Colonial Period, and a masterful hand at English prose, delivered in 1712 a Sermon,[11] in which he emphasizes the fact that sin is the cause of death. "Sin has been the Needle; Death has been the Thread."

This relationship is visualized in two senses, general and specific. Basically, of course, the sin of Adam is first conceived as bringing the penalty of death into the world. Mather, however, also relates sin to the individual case, in the following significant passage: "Some Sins there are that Naturally do Quicken the pace of Death. By intemperance men shorten their Lives. The Lewd Livers themselves do call it *Living Apace*. The Intemperate and Immoderate are but Short-lived; a *Short-Age* their Portion! In Excessive Eating, Men dig their own Graves with their Teeth. In Excessive Drinking, men Drown their Despised Lamp. Intoxications are Suffocations. By Unchaste Excesses, men extinguish their Brightness in a Premature Snuff of Rottenness. Excesses of Grief and Care, and Labour, do work Death."

When it came to the explanation of the outbreak of a special epidemic in a particular locality, however, the theory of the Wrath of God was not easy to apply. The Boston preacher, in referring to the current epidemic in Waterbury, Connecticut (called by Webster "putrid pleurisy"), says: "We do ourselves indeed, Enjoy a very great measure of Health; for which we owe all possible Thanks unto the God of our Health; and our Thanksgivings are to be quickened by what we see befalling others, that are not Greater Sinners than ourselves. But we ought Exceedingly to Sympathize with our dear Brethren, in an adjacent colony; where many have been Sick and Weak, and some Sleep."

Caulfield cites a broadside published in Boston during the 1735-1736 outbreak "On the prevailing Sickness, in many Towns in New-England with an earnest Call to Young and Old, to turn from Sin, and to seek God's Face and Favour,"[4] which contains the following verses:

"For God above, in Righteousness,
    An Angel sent with Power,
Who with a Sword already drawn
    Our Children to devour.

"What tears apace, run from our Face,
    to hear our Children crying
For help from pain, but all in vain,
    we cannot help their dying

"New England's Sins have greater been
    Than Sins of Heathen round,
Such breach of Laws, is the Grand Cause,
    God's judgments do abound."

The theory of the Wrath of God was again well expressed in 1737, by John Brown.[3] This clerical author begins with a complete statistical analysis of the Haverhill "throat distemper" tabulated by six-month periods and age periods. There were 256 deaths between November, 1735, and December, 1737, of which 210 were in children under 10 years of age, a very high incidence for a small community. The bulk of the volume is taken up by what might be called spiritual case histories of the pious and moving remarks made by the victims on their death beds. The children, themselves, were regarded as fortunate in being translated to Heaven with such sentiments on their lips. For the parents, however, the lesson of the epidemic was one of needed repentance. "Let us Cherish," he says, "and impress on our Hearts the Warnings and Admonitions we have received by the Sickness and Death of our Children, more tacitly or by their Mouths more expressly. Did not the very Circumstances of their Sickness and Death in itself, bring to Remembrance some of our Sins, and give us very bitter Reflections, on the Account of them? Either our careless Life in general, or some particular Faults; our not bringing them to Baptism, or neglecting to instruct them setting a bad Example before them, fond Indulgence or Unkindness toward them and passionate Treatment of them? And while we felt the hand of God so sorely correcting us therefor, were not we sorry and ready to wish for and promise Amendment of Life?"

To illustrate the persistence of this particular epidemiological theory, we may quote one more example from the last decade of the century. As Cotton Mather had preached in Boston about pestilence in Connecticut in 1712, so a Scotch Presbyterian minister in New York, 1793, discussed the scourge of yellow fever in Philadelphia. The Rev. J. M. Mason[10] told his congregation that the Lord had used the Revolutionary War, the domestic chaos following it, plagues of destructive insects, and Indian frontier attacks as preliminary warnings of the need of repentance. Now, in Philadelphia, "In all directions, fly the shafts of this unerring archer. Every day he multiplies his triumphs. The young, the old, the honorable and the vile, fall the indistinguished prey of this remorseless tyrant. Vain, as yet, have been all human expedients to arrest his progress, and baffle his power. He mocks opposition— he strews the earth with slain—He numbers among his victims even the 'masters of the healing art.' " Mason, like Mather, finds it difficult to discern why the Lord punished one city and not another. He continues: "Let none consider this dire calamity as an event in which only the immediate sufferers are concerned. To punish their iniquities it has doubtless been sent. But are they *single* in transgressions? Have *we* escaped because we are better than they? No, in no wise. A sovereign God has made them an example of his righteous vengeance. The evil under which they languish, is one of those awful dispensations by which Jehovah speaks, in thunder to a guilty people. The destroying Angel who is now executing upon our fellow citizens and fellow sinners the awards of Heaven, looks terribly on *us,* looks terribly on *all.* Whether he will bend his course hither God only knows."

MEDICAL APPROACHES TO EPIDEMIOLOGY

In considering the somewhat meager approaches to more naturalistic theories of epidemiology, it is important to realize the relatively retarded status of both medical theory and medical practice in the colonies prior to 1750.

Medical care was actually provided in these days by four different classes of practitioners. The first of these groups—and perhaps the most important in the Seventeenth Century—included the governors and other administrative officers, and particularly the clergy, who rendered medical aid to their people simply because they were the only persons in their communities who had any substantial basis of education. So, today, the leader of an exploring expedition in a remote area carries a first-aid kit and meets emergencies as best he can. The first representative of my own family on this continent, Governor Edward Winslow of Plymouth, administered "a confection of many comfortable conserves" to Massasoit, Chief of the local Indian tribe and—as was believed—cured him of a serious illness. The friendship, thus gained, was of basic importance in saving the little colony from a contemplated Indian massacre. Governor John Winthrop, Jr., of Connecticut (1606-1676), is said to have possessed a library of more than 1,000 volumes. "The scarcity of physicians in the colonies and Winthrop's willingness to give advice free of charge" caused him to be widely consulted. Cotton Mather says, "wherever he came, still the diseased flocked about him, as if the Healing Angel of Bethesda had appeared in the place."[7] In a later day, the combination of theology and medicine continued to be common. Jared Eliot (1685-1763) of Connecticut is a good example. Gordon[7] says of him that he "primarily devoted his life to the practise of the healing art. Toward this end he was an avid student, and he drank deeply from the well of Hippocrates, Galen and Celsus. He had a large following and since his success in the treatment of chronic ailments was great, he was called often to visit patients in every part of the Colony. He was the personal friend and correspondent of Berkeley and Franklin and the instructor of several medical students. It is related that in forty years he preached every Sunday and devoted at least some part of every week to the practise of medicine."

A second group of practitioners were the physicians trained in England or on the continent who came to the Colonies, as immigrants or as temporary visitors. They had often good fundamental training (of the limited type then available); but of those who actually stayed in the Colonies, few, if any, attained notable distinction. It is obvious that no successful English physician would be likely to settle in so remote an area. Colonials who went to Europe for medical training were very few in number prior to 1750.

A third group, and by far the most important in the early Eighteenth Century, were local men who had received apprentice training with older practitioners or had gradually built up a reputation by developing practice on their own initiative. Thus, Zabdiel Boylston (1679-1766), to whom we shall shortly refer in greater detail, was trained by an older physician, John Cutter of Boston. At first, of course, there were no barriers to practice; but in the Seventeenth Century, many Colonies passed licensure laws. Virginia took this step in 1639 and Rhode Island in 1641, for example.

Finally, of course, then as always, there were the quacks and charlatans. Gordon[7] quotes a historian of New York who said shortly before the Revolution, "Few physicians among us are eminent for their skill. Quacks abound like locusts in Egypt, and too many have recommended themselves to a full and profitable practice and subsistence. This is the less to be wondered at, as the profession is under no kind of regulation. Loud as the call is, to our shame be it remembered we have no law to protect the lives of the King's subjects from the malpractice of pretenders. Any man for his pleasure sets up for physician, apothecary and chirurgeon. No candidates are either examined or licensed, or even sworn to fair practice."

Shryock[17] sums up the case, as follows: "In the English-American colonies, medicine sunk gradually below the European level, and became largely a matter of 'kitchen physick' or of duplications of the remedies of Indian 'medicine men.' "

There was, however, in the early Eighteenth Century, one real advance in medical practice, the introduction of inoculation against smallpox by Zabdiel Boylston of Boston in 1721. He had almost died of smallpox himself in 1702; and, when the 1721 epidemic began, he and Cotton Mather had learned of the success of the new procedure in England and Boylston courageously began the practice. A veritable storm of opposition broke out. While a nephew was convalescing in Mather's house after inoculation a mob broke in and hurled a bomb (which luckily did not explode) into the patient's room. Conservative physicians organized a "Society of Physicians Anti Inoculator." Mather says he "never saw the Devil so let loose. . . . A lying Spirit was gone forth at such a Rate, that there was no believing any Thing one heard. . . . The People who made the loudest Cry . . . had a very Satanic Fury activating them. They were like the possess'd People in the Gospel exceeding fierce."

Increase Mather (then 83 years of age) and his son Cotton joined in publishing a single sheet folio statement in favor of Inoculation in which they cited the favorable results of this practice in the Levant, its success in England (including the patronage of the Royal Family) and the notable results of Boylston's inoculation of over 100 persons in Boston. Kittredge, in an introduction to a reprinting of the Mather statement, says, "In the history of preventive medicine, Zabdiel Boylston and Cotton Mather divide honors. Neither could have accomplished anything without the other."[15]

While it is true that inoculation was later regulated or prohibited by many colonial legislatures on account of the danger of spread of virulent smallpox by those who had themselves been inoculated, this episode marked the one outstanding example of the application of the experimental method in medicine on this continent. In this respect it was an event of major significance.

In general, however, it is obvious that the colonial physician, prior to 1750, could contribute little in the advancement of basic medical science. The difficulties in securing material for the study of human anatomy were practically insuperable. Dissection of cadavers was not legalized in this country until Massachusetts passed the first law which permitted it in 1831. Shryock[17] points out that physiological experimentation on the human body was also held unthinkable. He adds, "Imagine Galileo's difficulties, had the local mores prohibited the profane handling of pendulums and falling bodies." All that the physician could do was to report on his own clinical experience, and since that experience had no scientific basis, the results were rarely enlightening. A number of the early physicians were fairly good botanists for their day, and did add original observations on that science. Otherwise, what the colonial physician knew, aside from his haphazard experience, was what he derived from the classical authorities. If he possessed a copy of Galen or Avicenna or Vesalius, he was a fortunate man and a scholar. We can make our best guess as to what the best qualified of the early colonial physicians thought about epidemiology by considering the available body of knowledge at his disposal.

It is very doubtful if such a physician had ever heard of Fracastorius who advanced the concept of contagion so effectively in 1546; or of Kircher who urged a germ theory of plague in 1658; or of Leeuwenhoek who described bacteria in 1658. He probably did know that certain diseases were definitely contagious. Galen had listed ophthalmia, skin diseases, phthisis, and plague in this class. Avicenna included also variola, "pestilential fever" and others not readily identified. In the first of the plague tracts, Jacme d'Agramont in 1347[22] gives the list as "leprosy or scabies, phthisis and ophthalmia, pestilential fever, smallpox and measles and skin diseases." It is probable that "phthisis" in these early writings referred to influenza and not to tuberculosis. Of the important epidemic diseases, then, influenza, measles, and smallpox were no doubt regarded as contagious in the Seventeenth Century.

Probably the most deep-rooted philosophical concept of the period with regard to the causation of any unusual prevalence of disease was, however, the "epidemic constitution of the atmosphere." A peculiar condition of the air is the major cause to which Hippocrates attributed the epidemic diseases; and contagion is nowhere mentioned in the surviving portion of his writings. Thomas Sydenham (1624-1689)—"the English Hippocrates," the most influential figure in world medicine in the Seventeenth Century—closely followed his great predecessor in this respect. In his Collected Works, a careful analysis shows only three references to contagion, clear and definite with respect to plague and venereal disease, and incidental in his discussion of "intercurrent fevers." Contagion is not even mentioned in connection with smallpox and measles and not a single suggestion is made as to isolation procedures. Sydenham's emphasis (aside from the internal humoral status of the body) is almost wholly on (a) the influence of the known factors of climate and season, heat, cold, moisture, and dryness; and (b) the mysterious epidemic constitution of the atmosphere characteristic of a given year. Sydenham's contribution to clinical medicine was of the first importance and fully justifies all the admiration which was lavished on him; but "his almost complete neglect of contagion as a practical factor in the spread of epidemic disease and his major stress upon the metaphysical factor of epidemic constitution held back epidemiological progress for two hundred years."[24]

A more balanced analysis of the situation is to be found in the *Discourse on the Plague* published by Richard Mead in 1720; but this pamphlet had a much more restricted influence than the works of Sydenham. Mead was primarily a contagionist and lays down excellent rules for isolation and disinfection of fomites. Furthermore, when he considers the atmospheric conditions associated with prevalence at a particular place and time (which, in the light of existing knowledge had to be recognized) he stresses not the influence of the stars but the corruption of the atmosphere by local organic decomposition.[24] This factor had been commonly postulated by many earlier writers. Thus Jacme d'Agramont specifies that one of the reasons for prevalence of pestilence in a particular town is "filth, because to prevent pestilence in a town one must take vigorous steps to avoid the throwing out of entrails and refuse of beasts, or dead beasts near the town. Nor should manure heaps be placed inside the town. Nor must it be permitted that inside the town, in the streets, either in daytime or nighttime, any excrement be deposited or thrown out nor must there be kept inside the town skins to be soaked for tanning nor should cattle or other beasts be killed or butchered as has happened. From all such procedures great infection of the air occurs, in Paris, in Avignon and in Lerida."[22] Mead is even more explicit on this point. In explaining a local epidemic constitution of the atmosphere, he says, "It has besides been remarked in all Times, that the Stinks of *Stagnating Waters* in hot Weather, *putrid Exhalations* from the Earth; and above all, the Corruption of dead *Carcasses* lying unburied, have occasioned *infectious Diseases*."[24]

The concepts mentioned are common in all the medical literature of the time; and we may assume that the cultivated and well-

read physician of 1750 recognized five primary factors as governing the presence of epidemic disease, as follows:

1. (If he were a reasonably devout believer), the desire of God
to punish and warn his erring children.

2. The influence of climate and season (in the tradition of Hippocrates and Sydenham).

3. A mysterious epidemic constitution of the atmosphere characteristic of a given year (often associated with influence of the
planets and various abnormal natural phenomena).

4. A harmful influence on the constitution of the atmosphere of
a particular locality, due to organic decomposition.

5. Contagion (particularly in diseases such as influenza, measles
and smallpox in which case-to-case transfer was obvious and inescapable).

SANITATION AND QUARANTINE

Our forefathers were practical folks; and with a sound instinct,
they selected the last two of the factors listed in the preceding paragraph as actually promising the possibility of effective control.

The pastors and the governments which they dominated applied
their own epidemiological approach to the factor of Divine wrath
by days of fasting and of prayer. Like Oliver Cromwell, however,
they said, "Put your trust in God; but mind to keep your powder
dry."

The second and third primary factors mentioned at the end of
the preceding section did not lend themselves to practical preventive measures. "We all talk about the weather but no one
seems to do anything about it." Nor can we control the stars in
their courses. This was why Sydenham's emphasis on these factors had so fatalistic an influence.

The lay public, however, took seriously the fourth concept of
early medical writers which related disease prevalence to organic
decomposition; and special legislation against gross nuisances was
enacted in very early days. In England, as early as 1297, we find
legal regulations, requiring every man to keep clean the front of
his own tenement. In France, in 1350, King John II established
the first Sanitary Police in an ordinance which provided that hogs
should not be kept in cities; that streets should be cleansed, and
the offal removed; that butchers should not sell meat more than

two days old in winter, and one and a half in summer; and that fish should be sold the same day they were caught. In England, in 1357, a Royal order, addressed to the Mayor and Sheriffs, tells how the king, Edward III, passing along the river, had "beheld dung and laystools and other filth accumulated in divers places in the said city upon the bank of the said river" and had "also perceived the fumes and other abominable stenches arising therefrom; from the corruption of which, if tolerated, great peril, as well to the persons dwelling within the said city as to the nobles and others passing along the river, will it is feared arise, unless indeed some fitting remedy be speedily provided for the same." In the Court Rolls of Stratford-on-Avon in 1552 is found an entry that Shakespeare's father was fined for depositing filth in a public street, and he was disciplined again in 1558 for not keeping his gutters clean.[23]

In the American colonies, the same conception led to primitive but well-meaning attempts at control of disease by sanitation. Regulation of nuisances seems to have been entirely in the hands of local town authorities throughout most of the Seventeenth Century. Search of local records would, no doubt, reveal many instances of special orders in regard to sanitation. Action on a wider basis, according to Tandy,[18] began in South Carolina, where, in 1692, the provincial legislators enacted a regulation which forbade the running of swine at large in the streets of Charleston and directed all persons to cut the noisome weeds in and about the lots and streets. Later in the same year, the general assembly of Massachusetts empowered the selectmen and two justices of Boston, Salem, Charlestown and other market towns to assign locations for slaughterhouses and places for the trying out of tallow and the currying of leather.

The original charters granted by William Penn to Philadelphia and Chester in 1701 gave the mayors and magistrates power to cause the removal of nuisances. Obviously, amenity was a primary motive in such legislation. The control of disease was, however, specifically mentioned in a South Carolina provincial statute of 1704 which stated that, because of the filth of garbage and the nuisance of slaughterhouses, "the air is greatly infected and many maladies and other intolerable diseases daily happen." Similarly, a Massachusetts statute states that "by reason of the increase of said towns and places assigned for the use of noxious trades had become offensive and tended to breed infection."

Finally, the control of the fifth factor, contagion, was the object of much early legislative action. There was, of course, ample precedent here. The pandemic of leprosy which reached its height in Northern Europe in the Thirteenth Century was met by the construction of thousands of isolation camps or leprosaria and the control of this disease (whose actual etiology is still somewhat a mystery) was apparently successful. In the Fourteenth Century came the "Black Death," a major pandemic of plague; and here, too, isolation hospitals—and, particularly, measures of maritime quarantine—were applied on a vast scale. In 1374, Venice denied entrance to the city of infected or suspected ships, travelers or freight; in 1377, Ragusa rejected all travelers from plague districts who had not sojourned for a month at one of two designated points without developing the disease; in 1373, Marseilles erected her first quarantine station at which, after rigid inspection of the vessels, all travelers from stricken or suspicious ships were detained for forty days, and cargoes, ships and rigging exposed to elaborate processes of disinfection and to the influence of air and sunshine.[6]

No doubt the records of colonial towns would show evidence of action along the lines of quarantine procedure fairly early in the Sixteenth Century. The first instance known to the writer was taken in Boston in 1647 cited by General John Winthrop (father of Governor Winthrop of Connecticut, quoted on an earlier page) as follows: "For as much as this Corte is credibly informed that ye plagu, or like grieves infectious disease, hath lately exceedingly raged in ye Barbadoes, Christophers, and other islands, in ye West Indies, to ye great depopulating of those, it is therefore ordered, that all or other vessels coming from any pts of ye West Indies to Boston Harbor shall stop anchor before they come at ye Castle under ye poenalty of 100 pounds."[7] In 1663, when smallpox was prevailing in New York, the General Assembly enacted a law, of which the first sentence read: "This Court, understanding that the hand of God is gone out agaynst the people of New Netherlands, by pestilentiall infections, doe therefore prohibit all persons for comeing from any of those infectious places into this Colony, and amongst our people, until ye Assistants are informed and satisfied that the distemper is allayed."[21] In 1701, Massachusetts passed an act providing that when persons "were visited with the plague, smallpox, pestilential or malignant fever, and other contagious sickness," local selectmen were empowered to remove such persons to separate houses and provide nurses and attendants "at the charge of the parties themselves (if able)."[16]

In 1721, when Captain Joseph Allyn arrived at Wethersfield with smallpox aboard his sloop, the Governor and Council of the Connecticut Colony promulgated the following rigorous conditions for quarantine: "That the doors and windows of Mr. Allyn's house next the street, and at each end, be nailed up, and so effectually secured as to prevent anything being conveyed into or put out of the house on the side next the highway, or towards the neighbouring houses at each end; and that care be taken to let in sufficient air on the backside of his house."

"That the tenders on the sick, or nurses, be charged that whatever they have occasion to bring out of the sick person's room and throw out of doors, be carried out some back way, and in some convenient place for that end buried, or covered over with dirt, to prevent the dilating of any ill scent in the air."

The most complicated of these quarantine cases was, however, that of John Rogers of New London who returned from Boston sick of the smallpox in October, 1721. No less than twelve different meetings of the Governor and Council were devoted almost entirely to the "stupidity and stubbornness" and the "unruliness" of the family and friends of Rogers who repeatedly broke quarantine. Finally two guards were appointed to lodge at neighboring farms and keep "watch and ward day and night, and by coming as near to the house of said Rogers as they may without danger of infection, labour to understand the state of the sick there" and to discover and prevent any communication between the sick family and the outer world. All dogs belonging to the Rogers' household or commonly resorting thither were ordered to be destroyed. Finally, even one of the tenders of those who were sick became infected with unruliness, if not with smallpox, and returned contrary to express orders to his home in Groton where he in turn had to be quarantined.[21]

These are but a few examples of an innumerable number which might be cited. They suffice to indicate that our ancestors made an earnest effort to control epidemic disease by the only two practical methods at their disposal: sanitation and quarantine. It is unlikely that such primitive methods of sanitation as were available accomplished any significant results. Isolation and quarantine practices, even though they too were primitive, probably did sometimes actually check contagion. Important progress, however, must await the fuller epidemiological knowledge of the future.

ENLIGHTENMENT COMES TO THE COLONIES

The Eighteenth Century marked one of the major turning points in the history of mankind. Shryock[17] points out that "The general intellectual climate of the later eighteenth century was in marked contrast to that of the earlier decades. From the point of view of scientific men, it became distinctly fair and warmer. Modern experimental science, having developed rapidly during the seventeenth century, came into its own in the eighteenth." . . . "The eighteenth century was not only the 'Age of Reason' it was also the era of the Enlightenment, of the *Aufklärung*. . . . The Middle Ages, with their despair of this world and their hope for perfection in the next, were at last replaced by an era which rather despaired of the next world, but looked forward to perfection in this. There have been reactions since 1800, it is true, in the name of piety, of beauty, and of romance;* but no general return to the prescientific outlook has persisted long. In a very real sense, the eighteenth century *Aufklärung* marked the advent of the modern world."

This new movement began to make itself felt in the colonies about the middle of the century. The American Philosophical Society was founded in Philadelphia in 1743; the American Academy of Arts and Sciences in Boston in 1780. The American colonies contributed at least two world-famous leaders of the new scientific movement, Benjamin Franklin (1706-1790) and Benjamin Thompson (1753-1814), who became Count Rumford.

Medicine had its share in the spreading vistas of the time. About the middle of the century, ambitious young Americans began to go to Europe, particularly to Edinburgh, to study medicine. Saffron[14] notes that in 1749 John Moultrie, the younger, of Charleston, S. C., successfully defended a thesis "De Febre Flava" in the medical school at Edinburgh, as "the vanguard of a long line of eighteenth century Americans to receive their medical degree from that flourishing institution." Hermann Boerhaave

---

*Cf. Sartre and T. S. Eliot, today.

(1668-1738) of Leyden was the spiritual leader of this school, most of the Edinburgh faculty having received their training at his hands.

In the field of anatomy, John Hunter (1728-1793) had some 13,000 specimens in his London museum. In physiology, Stephen Hales (1677-1761) was measuring blood pressure. Albrecht van Haller (1708-1777) at Göttingen, who had been trained at Leyden, carried on the Boerhaave tradition of exhaustive and objective physiological experimentation. The major influence of his work was an emphasis on the supreme importance of tension and relaxation of the neuromuscular system of the body. John Brown (1735-1788) in Scotland carried this concept to an extreme in the "Brunonian system" of medicine, which had a determining influence on Rush and other leaders of American thought throughout the century.

The young American physicians, returning from their training in Europe, brought a new and fruitful inspiration to their careers in the colonies. Furthermore, they began to have real facilities to work with. The Pennsylvania Hospital, the first large and well-planned hospital in the colonies, opened its doors in 1751.

Local medical societies began to grow and increase their scope and influence. The New Jersey State Medical Society was founded in 1766, the College of Physicians in 1787. There was a rapid increase in such societies after 1790, and a corresponding growth of medical literature. The "Medical Repository" established in 1797, became one of the most important of American medical journals.

Most significant of all perhaps was the establishment of our own colonial medical schools, at Philadelphia in 1765, at New York in 1768, at Boston in 1783 (now the schools of the University of Pennsylvania, Columbia, and Harvard, respectively). Here our young men could be trained without a long voyage across the seas. Here the philosophy of health and disease could be taught. Here basic research could ultimately be planned and carried out. The "Healing Art" was becoming the "Science of Medicine."

YELLOW FEVER—THE AMERICAN PEDAGOGUE

Diepgen says of the Black Death in Europe, "A more frightful teacher than the plague, which swept over humanity with special fury in the middle of the Fourteenth Century, it is difficult to imagine." It was yellow fever which dominated American thinking about epidemiology in the late Eighteenth Century.

There were, of course, many epidemics of other diseases in the colonial period and in the early days of the republic. Chadwick or Webster, or both, cite epidemics of dysentery in 1751; of "Pepperill Fever" (perhaps typhus) in 1755; of influenza in 1756-1757, of measles and dysentery in 1759-1760; of diphtheria in 1773 and 1775; of dysentery in 1776; of influenza in 1781; of scarlet fever in 1783; of rabies in 1785; of measles in 1788-1789; of scarlet fever and smallpox in 1792; of "malignant typhus" in 1796; but none of these caused the terror or stimulated the scientific study associated with prevalence of yellow fever in the seventeen-nineties.

Yellow fever, according to La Roche,[9] appeared in Barbadoes in 1647 and was apparently first clearly described by Ferreyra da Rosa in 1694. During the last half of the Seventeenth Century it spread rapidly through the Caribbean area. It reached France in 1694; but its first clear descriptions in the North American continent were in Philadelphia, where it killed one-sixth of the inhabitants in 1699. It was introduced at Charleston in the same year and also in 1703, 1728, 1732, 1739, and 1740. Philadelphia had epidemics in 1741, 1747, 1748, and 1762; and other ports were also infected. John Mitchell wrote a monograph on yellow fever in Virginia in 1737, 1741, and 1742. John Lining wrote an account of the epidemic at Charleston in 1748.

After the seventeen-forties, epidemics of yellow fever in the North American continent were for a time rare (or undescribed). In the last decade of the century, however, there was a sudden outburst of activity; and Webster, following the general concepts of Sydenham, believed that this was the result of an epidemic constitution of the atmosphere that began to manifest itself in the measles of 1789 and the scarlet fever of 1792.

There was yellow fever in New York in 1791 and in Charleston in 1792; but the major storm broke on Philadelphia in 1793. La Roche[9] estimates that of a total population of about 50,000, there were 11,000 persons attacked, of whom some 4,000 died. Matthew Carey[5] says, "It is not probable that London at the last stage of the plague exhibited stronger marks of terror than were to be seen in Philadelphia from the 24th or 25th of August till pretty late in September." He tells us that few went abroad without protecting themselves by the constant application to their olfactory nerves of handkerchiefs or sponges, impregnated with vinegar or camphor. Some were found carrying pieces of tarred rope in their hands or pockets, or camphor bags tied about their necks. Many never walked on the footpath, but took to the middle of the street to avoid being infected in passing houses where deaths from the disease had occurred. Acquaintances and friends avoided each other in the streets, and contented themselves with a cold nod. Shaking of hands fell into disuse, and cases of persons shrinking back with affright at even the offer of the hand are recorded. A craped hat, or any other token of mourning, was carefully shunned; and many persons valued themselves on the skill and address with which they gained the windward of those they met and all uniformly and hastily shifted their course at the sight of a hearse.

In 1794, Philadelphia suffered a recrudescence of the disease, although in much less serious form; and New Haven had a small outbreak. In 1795, New York and Baltimore and Norfolk had their turn; in 1796, New York; 1798, Boston; Philadelphia suffered epidemics in 1797, 1798, 1799, 1802, and 1803. That of 1798 was almost as severe as that of 1793. All in all, this dread disease visited the North American continent 35 times between 1702 and 1800.

The serious outbreaks of a peculiarly devastating disease in our major seaports had one very interesting practical result—the creation of the first organized local health departments in this country. Special committees had, of course, been frequently appointed to deal with temporary emergencies. Such committees were appointed in Philadelphia and in New York in 1793; these tentative steps were followed by the creation of permanent boards of health, in 1794 and 1796, respectively. In 1797, state legislation was passed specifically authorizing the establishment of such boards by New York and Massachusetts. Huntington Williams[2] has, however, effectively supported the claim of Baltimore to the title of priority in this field. He offers evidence to show the following facts. The Laws of Maryland for 1893 contain an "Act to appoint a health officer for the part of Baltimore-town" (signed by the Governor December 28, 1793). John Ross and John Worthington had been acting as quarantine physicians since 1792, and it is apparent that they served under the Committee of Health which, prior to the state legislation, had been set up in September, 1793, and made a report to the citizens on the local absence of "the malignant fever" on September 14.

An additional quarantine physician for Baltimore was appointed in 1794. On January 1, 1797, Baltimore was incorporated as a city and promptly thereafter established a Board of Health as a recognized branch of the city government. This "Board of Health" became the "Department of Health" in 1900. There is apparently ample documentary evidence from the scrapbook and ledger of the Committee on Health to show that this Committee early in 1797 became the "Commissioners of Health" and that the use of the phrases "Health Department" and "Health Officer" indicate complete continuity from the first appointment of the Committee in 1793 to the establishment of the Board in 1797. Thus, there is here clear evidence of the creation of a permanent municipal body devoted solely, or primarily, to the public health. This body in Baltimore has had, since September 14, 1793, medical men serving officially as its agents and public funds at its disposal; and has been (with incidental changes in name) in continuous operation since that date.

For the purposes of the present discussion, we are concerned with the influence of yellow fever epidemics in the seventeen-nineties—not on public health administration—but on epidemiological thinking. This influence was far-reaching; and its significance may best be evaluated by the study of the contributions of the two outstanding figures in early American epidemiology, Benjamin Rush and Noah Webster.

BENJAMIN RUSH

Benjamin Rush (1745-1813) was undoubtedly the leading physician of his time on this side of the Atlantic. He studied at Edinburgh with Cullen and Monroe and in 1769 returned to Philadelphia to practice. He was at once appointed professor of chemistry in the College of Medicine, succeeded Morgan as professor of practice in 1789; and, in 1791, when the college became part of the university he was appointed to the chair of the Institutes of Medicine. He taught for 44 years and lectured to some 2,250 students.

One of Rush's major claims to distinction was his attitude toward mental disease. At the Pennsylvania hospital he was a pioneer in developing humane and scientific treatment of the insane. He was a blood-brother to the passionate and unrelenting—and often provocative—reformers of his day on the other side of the water, to Bentham, Cobden, Chadwick, Howard and the like. He campaigned for penal reform and against slavery and the use of alcohol and tobacco. He was an ardent patriot, a member of the First Continental Congress and a signer of the Declaration of Independence. During the Revolutionary War, he had a bitter quarrel with William Shippen, Jr., head of the medical department of the army, which led him even into sharp conflict with Washington. Yet at the close of his stormy life, John Adams could say of him, "As a man of science, letters, taste, sense, philososphy, patriotism, religion, morality, merit, taken all together Rush has not left his equal in America."

In medicine, Rush began as a disciple of John Brown, who had taken the somewhat extreme position (based on Haller's study of muscle-nerve functions) that all diseases were forms of two general physiological states, extreme tension or extreme relaxation. In his later years, Rush went even further, recognizing only one basis for disease—excessive "tension." The obvious remedy for all forms of disease was then relief of tension by purging or blood-letting; and Rush's extreme reliance on these measures caused bitter conflict with his confrères—and probably serious damage to his patients. Shryock[17] notes that at the time of his death Lettsome in London declared that Rush united "in an almost unprecedented degree, sagacity and judgment" so that he had astonished Europe; while Zimmermann in Hanover thought that all humanity should raise a statue to this American prodigy. Only thirteen years later, Elisha Bartlett was to observe of Rush's medical writings that, "in the whole vast compass of medical literature, there cannot be found an equal number of pages containing a greater amount and variety of utter nonsense and unqualified absurdity." Somewhat similar opposing conclusions could be drawn in respect to Rush's contributions to epidemiology—as viewed in 1813 and 1949; but a man can only be judged fairly in relation to the available knowledge of his time.

As early as 1787, Rush had published a paper on "bilious and remitting fevers," in which he relates what was presumably malaria to millponds and undrained areas, an acute piece of observation. It was the 1793 epidemic of yellow fever, however, which brought him into the thick of the fray; and his 400-page publication of 1794,[13] with several later pamphlets, dealt with this problem.

Rush was not concerned with the wrath of God, although the local preachers stressed this factor as usual. A Lutheran minister[8] pointed out with unction that "It was Philadelphia that imported from luxurious Europe the number of 70 or 80 actors and retainers of the stage, who actually arrived here exactly at the time when the fever raged with the utmost violence. It was Philadelphia that contained those parents who had given willingly 300 dollars to obtain a perpetual right of free access, with the wife and children, to the plays, in order to plunge themselves and their relatives the quicker into all kinds of dissipation, and obliterate in their hearts all taste for what is serious and useful."

Nor was Rush greatly interested in annual variations of the epidemic constitution of the atmosphere. He recognized the influence of season; but as a practical man, dealing with an epidemic in a particular section of Philadelphia at a given time, the problem which he faced was primarily a choice between contagion and local miasms.

Rush was one of the first to recognize the existence of the epidemic of yellow fever which he reported to the port physician on August 24. Throughout the terrible days when Washington had removed to Mount Vernon and nearly all federal and state and many city officials had deserted Philadelphia, he labored in the care of the sick with untiring devotion. He is said to have seen 100 cases a day and to have visited half the homes of the city. He himself was at last stricken down in October.

At the beginning of the outbreak, Rush, in his letter to the port physician calling attention to the seriousness of the epidemic, says, "whether it is propagated by contagion, or by the original exhalation I cannot say"; and in his 1794 publication, he keeps both factors in mind. This was much the same balanced judgment which had been expressed by Richard Mead in his classic report on the plague in London.[12] There was a profound difference in emphasis, however; Mead visualized local circumstances as favoring a primary contagion (much as we do today). Rush conceived a primary miasmatic influence which later culminated in contagion. "The exhalation infected at the distance of three or four hundred yards; while the contagion infected only across the streets." He mentions that "moschetoes (the usual attendants of a sickly autumn) were uncommonly numerous"; but this fact (with the presence of dead cats and the appearance of a meteor) is cited merely as supporting evidence of an unhealthy condition of the atmosphere.

The immediate crux of the controversy which soon developed was the relative importance to be attached to contagion and to local conditions. The College of Physicians on November 26, 1793, pronounced that "this disease was imported into Philadelphia, by some of the vessels which arrived in the port after the middle of July." They pointed out that "no instance has ever occurred of the disease called the yellow fever, having been generated in this city, or in any other parts of the United States, so far as we know: but there have been frequent instances of its having been imported, not only into this, but into other parts of North America."

Rush meets the importation theory with the following ingenious arguments. He points out that in the West Indies, yellow fever does not exist everywhere but is endemic only in those regions where marsh exhalations from vegetable putrefaction are present and when the force of these exhalations is intensified by hot and dry weather. The same causes (under like circumstances) must also produce the same effects. Therefore, since vegetable exhalations, in hot, dry weather produce yellow fever in the West Indies, the same causes must produce it in the United States. Putrefaction of damaged coffee on a wharf near Arch Street was the original cause of the 1793 epidemic.

From the beginning, there was a minority in the medical profession which vigorously opposed the theory of importation. John Redman, president and two other members of the College of Physicians, dissented from the 1793 report cited above, as did Dr. J. Hutchinson, the port physician. An active leader of the anticontagionists was the distinguished French physician, Jean Devèze. His opinion was based on direct observation of the Bush Hill Hospital set up in a suburb of the city for the care of yellow fever patients, where not a single new case of this disease developed among doctors, nurses and attendants in the most intimate contact with the disease. It is difficult to quarrel with this conclusion, in the light of existing knowledge. Yellow fever was *not* a contagious disease (in the absence of yellow fever mosquitos).

Rush was, in 1794, strongly opposed to the conclusion of Devèze that the malady was not spread by contagion (once its miasm had been generated by miasmatic decomposition). In his later writings, however, he moved into a more and more anticontagionistic position. When the epidemic recurred in 1794, 1797, 1798, and 1799, the old controversy continued. The College of Physicians still stressed importation and the doctrine of contagion was supported by the medical profession and the public as a whole; and in 1798 Rush wrote to Noah Webster, "Not more than twenty persons of any note believe the late epidemic was generated among us, and not more than fifty believe in its being generated at any time in the United States. The absurd idea of its being a specific disease is nearly universal in our city."

Rush, however, fought on and published three more pamphlets on the subject between 1799 and 1805 (reviewed in some detail elsewhere[24]). He concludes, categorically, that "This disease is the offspring of putrid vegetable and animal exhalation in all countries." He draws a suggestive contrast between two kinds of contagion. The first kind is "secreted as in the smallpox and measles in which state it acts uniformly, and without the aid of exciting causes, upon persons of all ages who have not been previously exposed to it." In other cases, as in the bilious fever, the contagion "is derived from certain matter discharged from the body which afterwards by stagnation, or confinement, undergo such a change, as to partake of the same nature as the putrid exhalations which produce the fever." This was a logical and sound distinction between diseases actually spread by direct contact of one human being and another and those which require an intermediate host (malaria, and yellow fever) for their transmission.

That yellow fever belonged to the second group was proved by the influence of season (the sharp cessation of an epidemic in cold weather) and by the fact that yellow fever "does not spread in the country when carried thither from the cities of the United States" and "does not spread in yellow fever hospitals when they are situated beyond the influence of the impure air in which it is generated."

These conclusions had a certain real validity. They were unfortunate in leading Rush to a more and more uncompromising opposition to quarantine measures. "Can the yellow fever be imported?" he asks in 1799; and replies, "I once thought it might but the foregoing facts authorize me to assert, that it cannot, so as to become epidemic in any city or country. As well might a coal of fire be brought from one of the West Indian islands to this country or a lump of ice be conveyed from this country to one of the West Indian islands, in the open air." Therefore he vehemently opposes all measures of quarantine, which he compares to an attempt to defend Moscow from the plague by placing an icon upon the city gate.

On the other hand, Rush had right on his side when he insisted on the values of sanitation. He was largely correct when he pointed out that yellow fever occurs only in hot and moist climates and seasons; and only in the presence of "marshes, millponds, docks, gutters, sinks, unventilated ships, and other sources of noxious air." Decaying coffee on the Arch Street wharf was not important, but Rush was correct in concluding that when certain local sanitary precautions were taken (precautions whose exact nature we understand, while he did not) "large cities shall no longer be the hotbeds of disease and death. Marshy grounds, teeming with pestilential exhalations, shall become the healty abode of men."

The College of Physicians saw one side of the shield; Rush and Devèze, the other.

NOAH WEBSTER

The epidemiological thinking of the Eighteenth Century came to its fruition in the work of another distinguished leader of post-revolutionary thought, Noah Webster.

Noah Webster (1758-1843) graduated from Yale and was admitted to the bar. He began his career, however, as a schoolteacher; and, with short intervals of law practice in Hartford and journalism in New York, his life was spent as a teacher and scholar, at Amherst, Mass., and New Haven, Conn. Early in his school experience, he began the preparation of a series of school textbooks on spelling, grammar, and reading. He was actuated in this work by a passionate patriotic desire to promote a specifically American culture, free from the domination of English thought; and his success was so great that 15,000,000 copies of the American Spelling Book were sold during the author's lifetime.[25] From these schoolbooks he passed on to a more formidable task, the preparation of a dictionary of the English language, based on American practice and adapted to American use. A dictionary for schools was published in 1806; but the *Magnum Opus* was completed in 1825 at Cambridge, England, and issued in New York in 1828. This was a monumental task, involving 12,000 words and 30,000-40,000 definitions not found in any previous dictionary. Furthermore, this was the first effort of its kind in which the methods of comparative philology were applied. Webster had a huge table built in the form of a hollow circle within which he worked with dictionaries in twenty languages ranged about him for reference and comparison. His firm and keen but kindly face still looks out at us from the frontispiece of current editions of this standard dictionary. The lineaments of no American of that time, except Washington, are so familiar to the American of today.

Webster's interest in epidemiology had been aroused by the influenza epidemics of 1789 and 1790, and the scarlet fever epidemic of 1793. The Philadelphia epidemic of yellow fever, followed by similar outbreaks in New Haven (1794) and in New York, Baltimore and Norfolk (1795) revived his curiosity "with double zeal." He sent out letters of enquiry to physicians in the cities concerned and in 1796 published a volume of essays and letters by ten physicians on experience in New York, New Haven, Sheffield, Mass., Norfolk, Va., Montgomery County, N. Y., and elsewhere.[20] Eneas and Elijah Munson in New Haven were contagionists; but nearly all the other authorities were miasmatists, particularly Valentine Seaman and Elihu H. Smith of New York. Webster, in summing up, sides strongly with the anticontagionist majority. Smith's analysis is the most balanced and most thoughtful of these communications. He notes that the question whether the yellow fever be "epidemic" or "contagious" is largely a question of terminology. If by the query whether disease is contagious "it is meant to inquire, whether the well become affected with the Fever, in consequence of the contact of a sick person or the clothing of a sick person, or from the performance of the offices of friendship, charity, and meniality, to those who were sick—I answer that no such cases have come to my knowledge." With regard to importation he concludes, "The whole, therefore, that can be granted, or ought to be assumed by those who maintain the disease which prevailed in New York in 1795, to have been imported is—That infection may be brought into any place (and therefore into this city) from abroad; that, under certain circumstances of the place, where it is introduced, it becomes very active and destructive; but that when these circumstances do not exist, however the person immediately affected—if it be introduced by a sick person—may suffer, it is harmless, so far as the general health of that place is concerned. If the subject were viewed in this light, as most assuredly it ought to be, the question of importation, or nonimportation, would sink into its merited insignificance; the efficient cause, the causa *sine qua non,* of such Fevers, would be clearly discerned as depending on local circumstances, capable of being wholly changed."

The preparation of this series of collected papers only whetted Webster's interest in the problem. He published a series of 25 letters to Dr. William Currie of Philadelphia controverting the importation theory and corresponded actively with Rush, who wrote that the letters to Currie "have made a greater impression upon our Citizens than anything that has ever been published in Philadelphia upon that subject." Finally, in 1799, Webster published a two-volume work on the Epidemic and Pestilential Diseases,[19] which admirably summarizes the state of knowledge of the time. The arguments of this book have been reviewed in some detail elsewhere[24, 25] and only their highlights can be touched upon here.

First, with regard to contagion. Following suggestions of Richard Bailey and Maclean of New York, Webster defines "specific contagion" as "a quality of a disease, which, within a suitable distance, communicates it from a body affected with it, to a sound body, with great certainty, and under all circumstances of season, weather or situation."[19] On the other hand, "That quality of a disease which may or may not excite it in a sound body within a suitable distance, or by contact; and which depends on heat, foul air, an apt disposition in the receiving body, or other contingent circumstances, and which may excite the disease in the same person more than once"[19] is given the denomination of infection.

Now the particularly interesting thing about this distinction is that Maclean and Webster cited measles and smallpox as examples of the first type, plague, dysentery and epidemic fevers as of the second. In other words, they recognized as contagious the two most common diseases due to filtrable viruses—the two in which neither well carriers nor infection by fomites is known. They even recognized the specially high degree of acquired immunity which characterizes these virus diseases.

In a later paragraph, Webster apparently transfers typhus fever from the miasmatic to the contagious class when he emphasizes "the necessity of distinguishing carefully between *epidemic* pestilence, proceeding principally from general causes in the elements, and marked by other epidemic diseases, by the failure of vegetable productions and by the sickness, or death of cattle, fish and other animals—and *diseases merely infectious,* generated by artificial means, which *may* be communicated, which may happen in jails, ships and camps, in the healthiest state of the elements, and which cease as soon as the infection can be dissipated by purifications and fresh air."[19]

For such maladies as yellow fever, however, Webster becomes more and more reluctant to allow any place for contagion. He is particularly bitter against Richard Mead. He says, "Dr. Mead's treatise on the plague has been much admired and celebrated yet I will assert, that next to the 'Traité de la peste,' a treatise in quarto on the plague of Marseilles, published by royal permission, it is the weakest and least valuable performance on the subject now extant." Yet, as a matter of fact, the *Traité de la peste* is an excellent bit of descriptive epidemiology; and Mead's *Short Discourse Concerning Pestilential Contagion* was probably the most significant contribution made since classic days, with the exception of the writings of Fracastorius. Webster's mind was, however, by this time absolutely closed to any suggestion of the importation of infection. He says, "In opposition to all these great authorities, it will probably be proved, that the plague generally if not always originates, in the country where it exists as an epidemic." He repeatedly heaps scorn on such "vulgar notions" as "that the plague is conveyed from country to country in bales of goods."

Commenting on the plague at Marseilles, he points out that there was a period of six weeks between a death from plague on the suspected incoming ship and the recognition of the disease in Marseilles, "a circumstance that renders it clearly impossible that there could have been any propagation of the distemper by infection." Until the roles of the rat and the flea were understood, this was a powerful argument. In the case of yellow fever at New Haven in 1794, he shows that the blankets from the schooner said to have produced infection had belonged to a sailor who had not been sick and had been kept by him in a chest and not used; while the blanket and clothing of the sailor who had died were carried to his home where they produced no disease. Without knowledge of the insect carrier, this is also good reasoning.

In general, Webster's arguments against contagion (in such diseases as plague and yellow fever) is based chiefly on the following arguments:

1. Cases occur without exposure to a pre-existing case of disease. Here, of course, was a perfectly sound argument. Webster is most effective in demolishing many detailed attempts of the contagionists to demonstrate actual routes of infection by fomites. He shows that at New Haven and Providence the blankets and clothing supposed to cause the primary cases could not have been infected and that the soiled blankets of an actual patient failed to produce results. He shows that the sufferers had generally not been in direct contact with previous cases and in certain instances had not been out of their houses for weeks. Until the role of the insect carrier was understood, such arguments were incontrovertible. A special case, under this general heading, is the point raised by Rush and Webster that the first case of a given disease must have arisen without prior contagion; and that, if this is so, later cases may arise in the same manner.

2. Direct exposure to cases of disease frequently—and, in the case of yellow fever, generally—fails to produce infection. The absence of secondary cases at the Bush Hill Hospital was Devèze's chief thesis, and the fact that patients from New York and Philadelphia who moved into the country never caused secondary cases was a powerful argument, definitely proving the necessity for some second factor, if it did not demonstrate the absence of any factor of communicability. A similar type of evidence was the failure of certain epidemics to spread from one community to another.

The localization of an epidemic in a particular area of a community is, of course, striking evidence that some factor other than contagion must be at work. So is the fact that epidemics run their course and then die out. If a chemical infection were the cause it should multiply in geometrical ratio until the human race were extinct. We explain this phenomenon partly by acquired immunity (which Webster denied in plague and yellow fever) and partly by seasonal influences. In the case of such a disease as influenza we assume a cyclical change in the virulence of the organism. But chemical infection as understood in Webster's day could hardly be supposed to show such a change.

Probably the most significant underlying factors which determined the reasoning of the late Eighteenth Century in regard to these problems were the current conceptions of the nonspecificity of diseases and of the nature of contagion. An important fact to bear in mind in connection with the epidemiological thinking of the time is that "contagion" was visualized as a chemical—not a biological phenomenon. Webster says, "Of the nature of the infecting principle in disease we know very little. . . . It is supposed that the diseased body discharges certain fine poisonous particles which are suspended and diffused in the air, and being imbibed by the pores of the skin and with the breath, excite the same species of distemper in a healthy body." The infecting principle in smallpox and plague must be very different, since the first always operates and the second only under certain circumstances. The infection in the case of plague and other autumnal diseases "appears to consist of a species of air, which is one of the elementary parts of all vegetable and animal substances. It may be what Dr. Mitchill denominates, the *septic acid;* that fluid which is discharged from flesh in the process of putrefaction. . . . It operates, in producing disease, no otherwise than all the morbid exhalations extricated from every species of vegetable and animal substances in the putrefactive process."[19]

"Webster and his contemporaries were, of course, perfectly sound in arguing that in the case of such diseases as the remittent and intermittent fevers, typhus, plague and yellow fever, the factor of infection as then understood could not possibly account for observed phenomena. To them, the theory of infection involved the simple assumption that (a) a previous recognized case of disease causes (b) a second recognized case of disease. This was often manifestly untrue. Today, we should say that either (a) a clinical case or (a1) a human carrier, sometimes plus (a2) an insect or animal carrier, or an inanimate carrier such as water or milk, causes (b) the second clinical case. It required knowledge of the germ and, particularly, of the human carrier to make the theory of infection plausible. This is why the medical profession, from Hippocrates to Pettenkofer and Murchison, fought against the laymen's fundamentally correct concept of communicability. The layman perceived the broad relationships; but the physician, knowing more, realized that there were fatal exceptions to any doctrine of communicability which could be formulated, until the role of the human and animal and inanimate carriers was understood."[24]

The second potential factor in the causation of epidemic disease was, of course, that of local miasms due to organic decomposition. "This was the factor commonly opposed to that of infection in the yellow fever controversies, and it was always recognized by Webster, although with varying emphasis. The fact that infection sometimes operated and sometimes failed to do so, the seasonal incidence of various diseases, and particularly the localization of epidemics in certain areas—usually low and waterlogged and uncleanly—pointed clearly to local influences. Webster considered such influences as determining with regard to the regular summer fevers (malaria, dysentery, typhoid, etc.) and as contributory in the greater pestilences (plague and yellow fever). He recognized the vicinity of marshes as of special importance, supporting this conclusion particularly with evidence from Italy and the United States where malaria was prevalent; and, in general, laid stress on dampness and accumulations of decomposing organic matter. Like Rush, he thought human and animal feces less important than decomposing vegetable and animal matter."[24]

"In the *Collection of Papers on Bilious Fevers* these local miasmatic influences received major emphasis, and here the reasoning of Webster and his contemporaries was essentially sound. They were quite right in believing that the infection of malaria and typhoid, of plague and yellow fever, would not spread unless local conditions permitted. In the greater part of the *Epidemic and Pestilential Diseases,* however, the factor of local miasms does not loom very large. Webster is chiefly concerned with proving the need for still a third factor, and emphasizes the fact that putrefaction and dampness and season often fail to produce the effects which would be expected."[24]

"This third factor—the one which Webster throughout the *Epidemic and Pestilential Diseases* chiefly emphasizes—is the general epidemic constitution of the atmosphere. From the time of Hippocrates, belief had persisted in such an influence, quite aside from local miasms, as accounting for the pandemic prevalence of the major plagues."[24]

"The epidemic constitution, according to Webster, was generally a world-wide condition and it was associated with other biological and meteorological phenomena of which the most important were epidemic diseases of cattle, fish, and other animals, diseases of plants, disappearance of birds who perceived and fled before the approaching calamity, plagues of noxious insects, storms, cold winters, hot summers, 'dark days,' floods, earthquakes, volcanic eruptions, and the appearance of comets and meteors. Such associations, or some of them, were accepted by the majority of medical writers from the days of the Greeks to the middle of the nineteenth century."[24]

Webster furnishes perhaps the most exhaustive summary of evidence upon this point ever collected. His volume 1 consists almost wholly of a year-by-year summary of epidemics and phenomena in the physical world which precede, attend, or follow them, from the Mosaic writings down to 1799; and volume 2 opens with the tabulation from 1650 down of yearly weather conditions, astronomical events and, volcanic eruptions in comparison with records from Bills of Mortality in various cities. Since out of 200 years covered, 67 show records of comets, 85 of volcanic eruptions and 179 of special prevalence of disease, the opportunities for coincidence are not inconsiderable.

It should be clearly emphasized, first, that Webster was not thinking of any mystical astrological influence but of a strictly physical one; and, secondly, that the various castastrophic phenomena listed were not supposed to cause each other but were all brought about by a deeper underlying condition of the atmosphere. "There must be an alteration in the chymical properties of the atmosphere to solve the difficulties that attend our inquiries into the cause of pestilence."[19] Webster was inclined to believe that the basic factor was electrical and associated with changes in the inner fires of the earth. Mephitic vapors might play a secondary role, but only electricity could account for all the mysteries involved; and Webster suggests that its influence on the human body may be exerted chiefly by producing excessive stimulation followed by debility.

It was this basic condition of the atmosphere which was the true cause of great pestilences; but its most terrible effects were produced only when reinforced by local miasms and were sometimes supplemented by infection. The cooperation of the three forces was easy to visualize. The epidemic constitution was a physical and chemical state of the atmosphere. Local miasmatic conditions added other deleterious chemicals (septic acid). Finally, contagion might contribute still other chemical effluvia of much the same nature, generated by the diseased body in its immediate vicinity, much as the local miasms were produced over a wider area in the neighborhood of marshes and accumulations of putrefying organic matter.

It must always be remembered that the student of 1799 was seriously handicapped by lack of any clear conception of the specificity of individual diseases. Rush, as we have seen, represented an ultra-Brunonian position on this point, assuming that all of what we now call "diseases" were forms of one basic malady. The whole trend of medical opinion was dominated by the views of Sydenham who taught that a particular epidemic at a particular time was a clinical entity; but that this entity was a unique one, produced by the influence of epidemic constitution and season on an earlier existing disease entity. Webster was entirely consistent with the best professional thought of his time when he said that "an epidemic disease—that is a disease due to the general epidemic constitution of the atmosphere—can be distinguished from one due to infection or specific contagion by two characteristics." First, it is always "preceded by influenza, affections of the throat or acute and malignant fevers." Second, it "predominates over other diseases; totally absorbing them or compelling them to assume its characteristic symptoms." "In every possible case, a plague that banishes other diseases, as I believe it always does, is an epidemic generated in the place where it exists; for it is not possible that this expulsion of other diseases could take place, unless the epidemic depended solely on the elements."

This was orthodox doctrine, deriving directly from Sydenham who described an epidemic of dysentery following smallpox which, "so nearly resembled the then reigning variolous fever that it would seem only the fever turned inwards, and fixed upon the bowels."[24] Again, he says that measles in 1670 and tertian fever in 1671 "prevailed so considerably as to overpower the smallpox, and prevent its spreading much. . . ."[24] La Roche,[9] in 1855 assumes a transition between the ordinary remittent and intermittent fevers and yellow fever. The specificity of tuberculosis was not accepted until Koch discovered the tubercle bacillus in 1882.

In such a fog of confusion, it is no wonder that the development of scientific epidemiology was long delayed; and it is perhaps a source of wonder that, under such circumstances, our predecessors made as much progress as they did.

THE STATE OF EPIDEMIOLOGY IN 1800

Until the development of modern medical science there was always a certain definite divergence between lay and professional attitudes toward epidemic disease. The general public, if devout, continued to invoke the theory of Divine punishment, in 1800 as in earlier periods. If more rationally minded, they clung, in spite of contrary medical opinion, to the theory of contagion. Knowing little of the complications of the situation but seeing that many people became ill at a given time and that epidemics actually spread from place to place (as in New Hampshire in 1735) they leaped to the sound conclusion that contagion must be at work and insisted on regulations for isolation and quarantine, as we have seen in earlier paragraphs; and in the last decade of the eighteenth century on the establishment of Boards of Health, primarily for purposes of quarantine. They saw only a part of the problem but they saw it correctly.

The physician and the philosopher, understanding more of the complexities of the problem (but not enough for its real solution), entertained theories which were, on the whole, less helpful than the instincts of the laity. These theories involved, as pointed out, three principles:

1. Contagion.
2. Miasms.
3. The epidemic constitution of the atmosphere.

Contagion was universally admitted in measles and smallpox and, with some qualifications, in typhus fever. In typhoid fever, dysentery, malaria, yellow fever, and plague, on the other hand, the physician gave contagion, if it existed at all, a very minor and secondary place; and this attitude continued until the dawn of the bacteriological era. La Roche,[9] in his classic monograph on yellow fever, published in 1855, devotes but thirty pages to facts and arguments in favor of the contagious character of the disease and 330 pages to "facts and arguments against contagion" and to "proofs of noncontagion." Even in 1898, an official bulletin of the U. S. Marine Hospital Service could say that, in yellow fever, "one has not to contend with an organism or germ which may be taken into the body with food or drinks but with an almost inexplicable poison so insidious in its approach and entrance that no trace is left behind."

It is true, of course, that the contagionistic theory of disease had been admirably stated by Fracastorius in 1546 and that Cardanus in 1557 and Kircher in 1658 had definitely advanced the concept of a "contagium animatum." Leeuwenhoek in the late seventeenth century had discovered and described bacteria and protozoa. Plenciz in 1762 had presented a profound analysis of the subject, in which he classifies malignant, pestilential, and petechial fevers, variola, measles, scarlet fever, camp dysentery, and the convulsive coughs of infants as both epidemic and contagious; rheumatic and intermittent fevers, as epidemic and possibly contagious; scabies, leprosy, elephantiasis, gout, venereal disease, rabies, and phthisis, as contagious but not epidemic. He maintains the independent entity of each of these diseases and concludes that the germs which caused them must be "worm-like," "animalculae" which "propagate and multiply," like the microbes described by Leeuwenhoek.

Such voices crying in the wilderness were, however, quite drowned out by the general trends of medical thought. Ackernecht[1] has recently presented an admirable review of the situation. He points out that throughout medical history, the pendulum has swung in cycles between the extremes of contagionism and anticontagionism. Richard Mead, in 1721, represented a peak of moderate contagionistic theory. But, Ackernecht[1] points out that "as a matter of fact, contagion and the contagium animatum were rather old theories around 1800"; and rather discredited theories. He adds: "It was, curiously enough, in the first half of the 19th century, that is, shortly before their final and overwhelming victory, that the theories of contagion and the contagium vivum experienced the deepest depression and devaluation in their long and stormy career, and it was shortly before its disappearance that 'anticontagionism' reached its highest peak of elaboration, acceptance and scientific respectability." He cites medical authorities in the 1840's who referred to contagion as representing the "remnants of childish ideas"; and as the exploded animalcular theory of Kircher and Linnaeus "which has hitherto been so feebly sustained by proofs, as to have at no time received general favor from the profession."

Ackernecht points out that the anti-contagionists were not blind reactionaries but were animated by the critical scientific spirit of the times. Their fight was—they believed—"against out-dated authorities and medieval mysticism; for observation and research against systems and speculation." He cites in detail the actual studies on yellow fever, on cholera, and on plague, between 1821 and 1867, which should be read by the student of this subject to realize how cogent were the arguments against contagion, in any form, in which a theory of contagion could be formulated in the light of existing knowledge. Furthermore, he points out the social and political factors involved which brought the arbitrary practices of quarantine into direct conflict with the interest of the rising mercantile class whose type of liberalism involved vigorous (and honest) opposition to interference with trade.

The fact was, of course, that no theory of contagion could work (in malaria, yellow fever, cholera, and plague) without acceptance of the theory of a living biological causative agent (which remained an unproved assumption); and, particularly, without the concept of the insect vector and of the well human carrier. Rush and Webster were not behind the times. They were leaders in the current scientific thought of their day, in limiting contagion to such diseases as smallpox and measles where there was no extra-human stage involved.

The second major factor in the epidemiology of 1800 was the concept of local miasms due to organic decomposition. This factor was put forward by almost all authorities and was tacitly—although not actively—accepted by the public at large. They were quite right in perceiving that epidemics occurred chiefly in unsanitary surroundings. In malaria and yellow fever, references to marshes and millponds and other undrained areas are frequent. In the case of cholera and plague, other forms of insanitation, of course, played a major role. Decaying coffee did not produce yellow fever in Philadelphia in 1794; but stagnant water did. By emphasis on sanitation, the epidemiologists of 1800 made a real contribution to public health. The full application of this principle required knowledge of the exact nature of "insanitation"; but Edwin Chadwick was to show half a century afterward, that even without such detailed knowledge, sanitation could actually control disease.

A reasonably balanced theory, involving both the factors of contagion and local miasms could have led to a combination of quarantine procedures and sanitary reform which would have been fruitful in its results; and such a program might have been possible in the climate of the early attitudes of Rush and Webster. Unfortunately, both of them were driven by their opposition to contagion as a sole cause into denial of any significance at all in what the public, dimly, but correctly, defined as a real factor in the situation.

Contagion (or rather, infection) and local insanitary conditions could, in combination, explain why disease prevailed in a particular area at a given season. The reason why it occurred in one year rather than another was a more difficult problem to solve. Ships from the West Indies came to Philadelphia in 1793 as in 1794. Why did the epidemic occur in one year and not in the other? It was here that the epidemic constitution of the atmosphere came in as a logically necessary factor.

Even in the Hippocratic writings, while that sound empiricist laid main stress on the human constitution and on climate and season he does call in the "epidemic constitution of the atmosphere" to explain the residual phenomenon of unusual prevalence of epidemic disease. Most authors of the plague tracts did the same, in the 14th century, the Paris faculty of medicine being quite convinced that a conjunction of Mars, Jupiter, and Saturn, in the sign of Aquarius at one o'clock in the afternoon of March 20, 1345, was the basic cause of the trouble. Even Fracastorius admits that "astrologers often predict that certain diseases and epidemics will arise" citing examples of such successful predictions. Kircher has a lengthy discussion of the influence of the constellations on plague. Sydenham, of course, made this factor basic in all his thinking. He does not take the stars into much account; but he says that "There are various general constitutions of years, that owe their origin neither to heat, cold, dryness, nor moisture; but rather depend upon a certain secret and inexplicable alteration in the bowels of the earth, whence the air becomes impregnated with such kinds of effluvia, as subject the human body to particular distempers, so long as that kind of constitution prevails."[17a] The theory of epidemic constitution, developed to the degree to which Sydenham developed it, provided an imposing verbal explanation of any phenomenon which might occur; but such a facile answer closed the door to research and made any real progress in epidemiology slow and difficult.

Webster followed Sydenham in his overwhelming stress on the epidemic constitution. He accepts the concept that in pestilential periods diseases gradually progress and develop from measles and influenza to diseases of the throat or anginas and finally to pestilential fevers in the summer. Such pestilential periods are generally world wide in their incidence. Influenza, in particular, is "evidently the effect of some insensible qualities of the atmosphere; as it spreads with astonishing rapidity over land and sea, uncontrolled by heat or cold, drouth or moisture. From these circumstances, and its near coincidence in time with the violent action of fire in earthquakes and volcanoes, there is reason to conclude the disease to be the effect of some access of stimulant powers to the atmosphere by means of the electrical principle. No other principle in creation, which has yet come under the cognizance of the human mind, seems adequate to the same effects."[19]

The reality of the factor of epidemic constitution was then almost universally accepted; but the degree of emphasis laid upon it varied widely. Men of a practical empirical turn of mind, such as Hippocrates and Richard Mead, admitted it as a possibility, but paid little practical attention to it. Even Rush emphasized miasms rather than epidemic constitution. On the other hand, logical theorists, like the members of the Paris faculty and Noah Webster, made epidemic constitution the cornerstone of their philosophy. It is perhaps surprising that Sydenham, with his wealth of direct clinical experience, should have become the leader and inspirer of this school. Yet the advocates of epidemic constitution were fully justified in raising a vital issue. There is still a basically unknown "X factor" in epidemiology.

We do not really know why influenza became pandemic in 1918 any more than the authors of the plague tractates knew why plague became pandemic in 1348. We guess that a variation occurred in the virulence of a living germ; this is only an assumption, backed by no concrete evidence. It is the most plausible assumption in the twentieth century; but could not have been postulated in the eighteenth. Our predecessors, working, as they inevitably did, on the basis of a theory of atmospheric corruption (of a chemical, not a biologic nature) and dealing with an effect which was often world wide and not local, naturally resorted to the celestial universe for an explanation. So we find the physician of the time turning to a malign conjunction of the stars as the ultimate cause of the phenomena which they were seeking to explain.

The practical man turned away from such a vague abstraction. Mead[12] says in regard to assumed atmospheric factors "It may be justly censured in these writers that they should undertake to determine the specific nature of these secret changes and alterations which we have no means at all of discovering." Webster[19] says in comment that this phrase is "very exceptionable as it is calculated to check a spirit of free inquiry, a spirit to which mankind is greatly indebted for improvements in science." Mead was right in challenging any theory, incapable of scientific proof or disproof. Yet Webster was also right. In his *Epidemic and Pestilential Diseases* he did apply a scientific test of the theory by comparing the relation of celestial phenomena to epidemic disease. His statistical procedures were crude and his conclusions erroneous; but the approach was sound. Accumulated experience and new scientific knowledge have demonstrated that the epidemic constitution was a gratuitous and untenable assumption.

We have still our "X factors" in epidemiology. We recognize them and we are studying them. The scientific renaissance of the Eighteenth Century, in which our own Franklin and Rumford and Rush and Webster played a not undistinguished part, laid the foundation for the achievements which have been won and those which are to follow. A study of their thinking may still help us to advance their achievements and avoid their errors.

References

1. Ackernecht, E. H.: Anti-Contagionism Between 1821 and 1867, Bull. Hist. Med. 22: 562, 1948.
2. Baltimore Health News 20: 193, Dec., 1943.
3. Brown, J.: A Relation of Some Remarkable Deaths Among the Children of Haverhill Under the Late Distemper in the Throat With an Address to the Bereaved, Henchman, 1737.
4. Caulfield, E.: The Throat Distemper of 1735-1740, Yale Journal of Biology and Medicine, 1939.
5. Carey, Matthew: A Short Account of the Malignant Fever Prevalent in Philadelphia, 3d ed., Philadelphia, 1793.
6. Eager, J. M.: The Early History of Quarantine, Yellow Fever Institute Bulletin No. 12, Public Health and Marine Hospital Service, Washington, 1903.
7. Gordon, M. B.: Aesculapius Comes to the Colonies, Ventnor Publishers, Ventnor, N. J., 1949.
8. Helmuth, J. H.: A Short Account of the Yellow Fever in Philadelphia, for the Reflecting Christian, 1794.
9. La Roche, R.: Yellow Fever, Blanchard and Lea, Philadelphia, 1855.
10. Mason, J. M.: Sermon on a Day Set Apart for Public Fasting, Humiliation and Prayer on Account of a Malignant and Mortal Fever Prevailing in the City of Philadelphia, S. Lowden, N. Y., 1793.
11. Mather, C.: A Sermon Occasioned by the Raging of a Mortal Sickness in the Colony of Connecticut and the Many Deaths of Our Brethren There, T. Green, Boston, 1712.

12. Mead, R.: A Short Discourse Concerning Pestilential Contagion, and the Methods to be Used to Prevent It, 2d Dublin ed., George Grierson, 1721.
13. Rush, B.: An Account of the Bilious Remitting Yellow Fever, as It Appeared in the City of Philadelphia in the Year 1793, T. Dobson, Philadelphia, 1794.
14. Saffron, M. H.: The Cultural Contributions of the Physicians in America (1750-1815), Dissertation Submitted for the Degree of M.A., Faculty of History, Columbia University, 1949.
15. Several Reasons Proving that Inoculating or Transplanting the Smallpox is a Lawful Practise and That it has been Blessed by God for the Saving of Many a Life, Reprinted for Private Distribution, With an Introduction by G. L. Kittredge, Cleveland, 1921.
16. Shattuck, L.: Report of the Sanitary Commission of Massachusetts 1850. Reprinted, Harvard University Press, 1948.
17. Shryock, R. H.: The Development of Modern Medicine, University of Pennsylvania Press, Philadelphia, 1936.
17a. Sydenham, T.: The Works of Thomas Sydenham, M.D., Translated by R. G. Latham, 2 vol., London, Printed for the Sydenham Society, 1848.
18. Tandy, E. C.: The Regulation of Nuisances in the American Colonies, Am. J. Pub. Health 13: 810, 1923.
19. Webster, N.: A Brief History of Epidemic and Pestilential Diseases, 2 vol., Hudson and Goodman, Hartford, 1799.
20. Webster, N.: (compiler), Collection of Papers on the Subject of the Bilious Fevers Prevalent in the United States for a Few Years Past, Hopkins, Webb and Co., N. Y., 1796.
21. Winslow, C.-E. A.: Development of the Public Health Movement in Connecticut. History of Connecticut, Ed. by N. G. Osborn, States History Co., N. Y., vol. V, p. 477, 1925.
22. Winslow, C.-E. A., and Duran-Reynals, M. R.: Jacme d'Agramont and the First of the Plague Tractates, Bull. Hist. Med. 22: 747, 1948.
23. Winslow, C.-E. A.: Evolution and Significance of the Modern Public Health Campaign, Yale University Press, 1923.
24. Winslow, C.-E. A.: The Conquest of Epidemic Disease, Princeton University Press, 1943.
25. Winslow, C.-E. A.: The Epidemiology of Noah Webster, Tr. Conn. Acad. Arts & Sciences 32: 21, Jan., 1934.

II. THE PERIOD OF GREAT EPIDEMICS IN THE UNITED STATES (1800-1875)

Wilson G. Smillie, M.D., F.A.P.H.A.*

THE first part of the nineteenth century in America was characterized by a series of great epidemics. They were initiated by the dreadful attack of yellow fever in the national capital of Philadelphia in 1793, and continued unabated for over half a century. These epidemics began to decline in extent, frequency, and virulence about 1870, and within a generation, they vanished completely.

Why did the nation suffer from these devastating plagues? What were the factors that were responsible for these disasters? Why did the epidemics disappear?

During the colonial period, there had been many epidemics, but they did not have the magnitude of the disasters of the following century. The greatest epidemic of all occurred among the Indians just before the settlement of the Pilgrims in Massachusetts Bay, devastating the savages to such an extent that they offered no resistance to the pioneers. During the prerevolutionary period, the colonists suffered severely, from time to time, from certain infections, particularly smallpox. One severe epidemic of septic sore throat[1] and scarlet fever swept over New England in 1735, taking a heavy toll of children and adults alike. Toward the end of the eighteenth century, yellow fever ravaged the port cities.

It seems probable that the colonists did not suffer from repeated, overwhelming epidemics because of their geography and social structure. They consisted of a pioneer population, living on scattered farms and in small villages. The population was quite stable; transportation was slow and difficult. A person was born and lived his entire life in the same house, often never leaving his village. There were no large cities, and there was relatively little contact with the outside world.

As indicated, the period of great epidemics really began in 1793, in the capital city of Philadelphia, then the second largest

*Professor and Chairman, Department of Preventive Medicine and Public Health, Cornell University Medical College, New York, N. Y.

city in America. It proved to be an outbreak of yellow fever which resulted in the death of nearly one eighth of the population. This epidemic has been described in detail by Philadelphia's leading physician, Benjamin Rush,[2] who attributed it to a pile of rotting coffee on Ball's wharf.

We can, best understand the epidemiological concepts of this whole period from a study of Rush's essay on *The Phenomena of Fever*. Epidemic diseases were called "zymotic" diseases from the

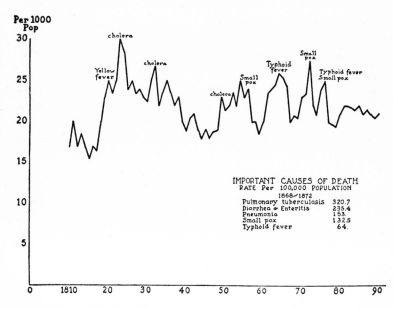

CRUDE DEATH RATE PHILADELPHIA 1810-1890
RATE PER 1000 Pop.

Graph 1.—Philadelphia was America's healthiest city, with a death rate of one-half or less than that of other large cities. The epidemic period lasted from 1820 to 1875. Cholera, smallpox, and typhoid fever were the tyrants, but the important causes of death were tuberculosis, and diarrhea and enteritis of babies.

Greek word *zymos* meaning "fermentation." These zymotic diseases were believed to be due to a fermentation of the tissues and always produced by an external stimulus. This stimulus often was cosmic in origin and was almost always transmitted through the air. The miasma might be produced by man himself, by the products of his household, or by any type of decaying vegetable or animal matter, or by cosmic phenomena. Zymotic diseases were always accompanied by fever.

The basic theory of Rush[2] was that, "There is but one fever. However different the predisposing, remote, or exciting causes of fever may be, whether from cosmic forces, marsh or human miasmata, there can be but one fever. Furthermore, there is but one exciting cause of fever, and that is *stimulus*. This proposition cuts the sinews of the division of diseases from their remote causes. Thus it establishes the sameness of pleurisy, whether it be excited by heat following cold, or by the contagion of measles or smallpox; or the miasmata of yellow fever."

Noah Webster,[3] who had a great influence on Rush's philosophy relating to epidemic diseases, published in 1799, his *History of Epidemic and Pestilential Diseases*. In this scholarly treatise of two volumes, he was able to show the relationship of cosmic forces, such as volcanic eruptions, showers of meteors, and other environmental factors in the production of serious epidemics and pestilential diseases. According to Webster, epidemics were due to an accumulation of special unfavorable environmental factors which combined to affect large numbers of people at the same time and thus produce overwhelming disaster. This extraordinary theory kept its firm hold on the minds of medical men for more than half a century.

A general summary of the opinion of the physicians who met at the Sanitary Conference of Paris in 1851 is illuminating. The conclusions of the Conference as presented by Clot-Bey[4] were:

1. Epidemics are always the result of cosmic conditions.

2. Isolated, e.g., individual, ill persons attacked by contagious diseases, virulent or miasmatic, are absolutely unable to produce epidemics.

3. Even epidemic diseases of essential contagious character are never spread through transmission, e.g., from person to person.

4. The essential, the specific, in epidemics is produced by a certain "state of affairs," unknown meteorological conditions, invisible and unfathomable.

The conference defined virulent diseases as variola, vaccinia, syphilis, and perhaps scarlet fever. Miasmatic diseases were typhoid fever, dysentery, cholera, intermittent fevers, and malaria. Plague, it was stated, did not fall in any group and thus could not be contagious.

Epidemiological concepts of this type did not require the isolation of the sick person, and quarantine was not enforced against individuals who arrived in a port upon a "sickly vessel," but against their effects, and against the ship's cargo. This theory is clearly expressed by the Quarantine Act of London of 1825,[5] and from the records of the famous Quarantine and Sanitary Convention of

CRUDE DEATH RATE NEW YORK CITY 1810-1890
RATE PER 1000 Pop.

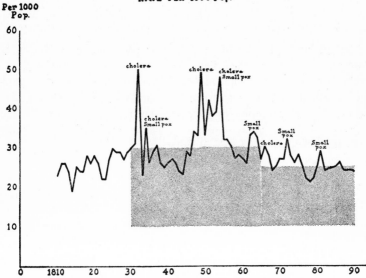

Graph 2.—The period of epidemics in New York City lasted from 1830 to 1880, then disappeared. Cholera and smallpox were the worst offenders, but the great "undertones of death," shown by the shading, were far more important and destructive.

1857,[6] called by Wilson Jewell of Philadelphia. This first convention was followed by similar conventions in 1858, 1859, and 1860. Their deliberations dealt almost exclusively with maritime quarantine and with environmental sanitation. The great debate of the 1859 Conference between Dr. Stevens and Dr. John Francis of New York on the resolution, "Personal quarantine of yellow fever may be safely abolished, since there is no evidence that the disease is contagious, that is, conveyed from one person to another," resulted in an overwhelming vote of the Conference that the individual with yellow fever is not dangerous to others.

It is clear that the average person of the street was not as firmly convinced as physicians were, that individuals with smallpox, cholera, and yellow fever were not dangerous to others. Thus the regulations of the lay boards of health of the period do concern themselves with isolation of the sick during epidemic periods, as well as with removal of dead animals and location of cemeteries.*

Medical science, however, held strictly to the dogma that zymotic diseases were not transmitted from person to person and that epidemics were due to natural phenomena, which were, for the most part, uncontrollable.

One is led to the conclusion that epidemics must, per force, prevail in a community which held such a tragically fallacious philosophy. Certainly these beliefs did not aid in the prevention or control of infectious diseases. However, we are willing to advance the theory that these fallacies were not entirely responsible for the prevalence of the great epidemics. With some temerity, we suggest that these epidemiological fallacies were not even very important factors in production of epidemics. The great epidemics during the nineteenth century were an integral, almost essential part of the development of the economy of the nation and the social structure was of a type which produced high death rates, with periodic disastrous epidemics almost inevitable. Furthermore, we shall show that the great epidemics disappeared, and the over-all death rates declined because of changes in social conditions. They declined before the causes of infectious diseases were known, before the epidemiological factors producing epidemics were understood, and before effective official health services were established.

What were the real causes of the great epidemics? What were the factors that produced, during that period, a higher continuous annual death rate in the American cities than the death rate of any other city of any civilized nation of the globe?

The great *epidemic peaks* of the crude death rate curve were caused by recurring invasions of Asiatic cholera, by smallpox, and

---

*J. H. Rauch of Chicago, in 1866, in a privately presented pamphlet, points out the great dangers of burial of those dead with contagious disease within the city limits. Burial should be far from populous places and at a depth beneath the surface sufficient to prevent contamination of the air.

in the seaports by yellow fever. Worst of all was cholera. The epidemic of cholera from 1845 to 1855 swept over the nation at the time of the California Gold Rush, with its great movement of population and pioneer expansion to the far West. Thousands and thousands of young, vigorous, hardy men, who started to California to make their fortune, left their bones on the plains along the western trails, struck down by cholera. Time after time, cholera invaded

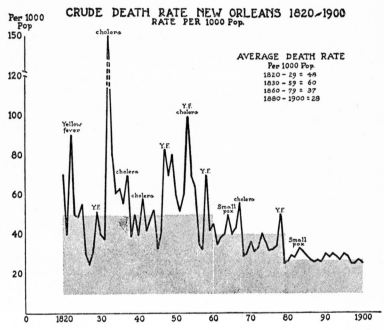

Graph 3.—New Orleans had a terrible mortality record, with a mean death rate of over 60 per thousand for more than thirty years. The epidemic period lasted from 1820 to 1880. Cholera and yellow fever were the worst offenders.

the ports of New York, Philadelphia, Baltimore, and New Orleans, swinging in ever-widening circles, to the smaller cities and to rural communities.

The epidemic disease that was dreaded even more than cholera was yellow fever. New Orleans fared worst of all the port cities, but none of these were spared from invasion, even as far north as Halifax. The disease, after invading New Orleans, would sweep up the Mississippi River to the interior towns, spreading terror as it came, but it never invaded the towns and rural areas that were removed from the main waterways. The situation became so serious that New Orleans, with its great wealth of natural resources had a much higher death rate than birth rate for nearly a century, and maintained her population only by the immigration of those hardy adventurers who were willing to take the great risk of their lives for the unparalleled financial opportunities offered by this fabulous city.

Smallpox recurred in epidemic waves and took a heavy death toll. Vaccination had been introduced in 1800, but was not widely accepted, and thus the disease always found ample susceptible material in the rapidly shifting, rapidly growing, unstable, pioneer community. We often forget the chief reason for the prevalence of smallpox in America during the nineteenth century. It is true that the cowpox vaccine was introduced in our nation by Benjamin Waterhouse in 1800, but *calf lymph* did not become available until 1870. The method of vaccination was from arm to arm, with all its attendant difficulties and dangers. Many outbreaks of syphilis occurred which were due directly to vaccination transmission.* Frequent transmission of erysipelas, and other virulent human infections, resulted from arm to arm vaccination, and thus the method of smallpox prevention was justifiably unpopular.

Negri of Naples, produced a good quality of calf lymph in 1834. The method was introduced into France by Lanoix in 1864 and to Prussia and Brussels in 1865. In 1870, H. A. Martin of Boston, distributed the first calf lymph in America, on dried quill points, for vaccination against smallpox. The method was not too successful for the dried vaccine soon lost its potency.

Although pestilential diseases of cholera, smallpox, and yellow fever were held in horror by the people, the real enemies which were producing the enormously high death rate caused little concern. These monstrous undertones of death were of everyday occurrence; for these diseases invaded every family, and their very familiarity brought about casual and inevitable acceptance.

The principal causes of death during the period of the great epidemics were not cholera, smallpox, and yellow fever, but were pul-

---

*In the Rialta, Italy, syphilis epidemic of 1861, 46 children and 20 nurses were infected with syphilis from an initial arm to arm vaccination.[7]

monary tuberculosis, diarrheal diseases of infancy, bacillary dysentery, typhoid fever, and infectious diseases of childhood, particularly scarlet fever, diphtheria, and lobar pneumonia.

Shattuck notes in his report of the Sanitary Commission of 1849,[8] that the most common infectious disease of all was malaria. It invaded every city, every town, every hamlet, and every home throughout the vast continent. As Boyd[9] has emphasized, malaria was the

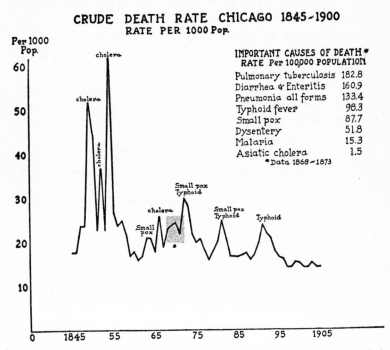

CRUDE DEATH RATE CHICAGO 1845~1900
RATE PER 1000 Pop.

IMPORTANT CAUSES OF DEATH*	
RATE Per 100,000 POPULATION	
Pulmonary tuberculosis	182.8
Diarrhea & Enteritis	160.9
Pneumonia all forms	133.4
Typhoid fever	98.3
Small pox	87.7
Dysentery	51.8
Malaria	15.3
Asiatic cholera	1.5
*Data 1868~1873	

Graph 4.—Chicago was a much younger city than the others. Its period of epidemics lasted from 1848 to 1890. Again, cholera, smallpox, and typhoid fever were the destroyers. A cross section of 1868 to 1873 shows that the important causes of death were tuberculosis, infant diarrhea, and pneumonia.

most familiar of all the fevers to our forefathers. It rose to its greatest height during the middle of the nineteenth century. It became somewhat stabilized in the eighteen fifties, only to break out with increased violence during the Civil War, and extended through the postwar recovery, well into the twentieth century.

"The extent to which Zymotic diseases prevail is the great index of public health," says Shattuck in 1849, "when the proportion is comparatively small, the condition of public health is favorable; when large, it is unfavorable."[8]

"But diseases of the respiration organs furnish one of the largest classes of causes of death. Consumption; that great destroyer of human health and human life, takes the first rank as an agent of death. It destroys $\frac{1}{7}$ to $\frac{1}{4}$ of all that die. The occasional visits of cholera or some other epidemic disease, creates alarm and precautionary means are adopted for prevention. But where is the alarm and precaution against a more inexorable disease over which curative skill has little or no power."[8]

An index of the supreme importance of tuberculosis as a cause of death is secured from the death records of some of the larger cities, where the rates of 350 to 400 per 100,000 population were the rule during the fifth decade of the century.

A report of the New York Sanitary Association in 1857[10] states that New York City had the highest death rate (36.8 per 1000 population) of any of the large cities in the world. The reasons for this were manifold. The city had increased very rapidly in population and harbored over 600,000 people. In the previous 12 years, a horde of immigrants had poured into the Port of New York—nearly 2,500,000 of them. Many of these poor people were destitute, starving Irish fleeing from their potato famine. They arrived without resources, in a terrible state of malnutrition and, crowding into the basement tenements under desperately filthy and foul conditions, they died in appalling numbers. Deaths from diarrheal diseases of infancy increased 250 per cent. Smallpox, typhus fever, cholera, even erysipelas and cerebrospinal meningitis swept through these wretched hovels, slaying the helpless victims by the thousands. In the first six months of the year 1858 alone, 425 persons died of smallpox in New York City.

The city had no sanitary protection whatever. It is true that the health inspector's office had been established early in the century, and there had been medical men in charge of these municipal functions until 1844. The department then fell into the hands of politicians. In 1858 the Board of Health consisted of the Mayor, Aldermen, and Councilmen. There was no Health Officer. Six Commissioners of Health were appointed by the Mayor, but their duties pertained to quarantine only, and they had no powers to regulate the sanitary condition of the city. There were merely twenty-two health wardens whose duty it was to supervise the sanitary conditions of the various wards. There was not a physician in the group. Instead, these wardens were an ignorant, vicious collection of ward heelers who had no knowledge of or interest in the health protection of the city.

CHANGE IN SEASONAL DISTRIBUTION OF DEATHS
UNITED STATES
1850 COMPARED WITH 1945

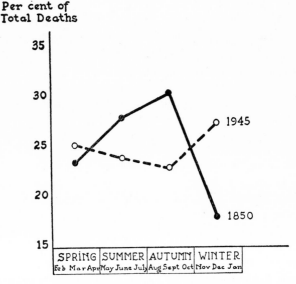

Graph 5.—One hundred years ago, autumn was the period of highest mortality and the winter months were most salubrious. Now, the situation is completely reversed.

Professor Dick of Nebraska, in the book *Sod House Frontier*[11] notes that in the 1850's on the western plains, cholera, typhoid fever, the ague, pneumonia, and smallpox were the prevailing diseases. Diphtheria took a heavy toll of children. Hardly a family escaped diphtheria, and in some instances whole families were wiped out. Water was obtained from springs, sloughs, water holes, and buffalo wallows. This supply was frequently contaminated. Water was scarce and hard to get. It was often necessary to dig two hundred feet to obtain water. In the early days there was no equipment for drilling and no pumps.

"A contributing factor to illness was lowered vitality from improper clothing, exposure and unbalanced rations. The common diet was salt pork, corn bread and dried foods. Settlers searched the fields for 'greens' and used weeds of all sorts to supply their vitamins."

"Malaria," says Dick, "was the disease of the young, and caused more deaths than any other illness. Pneumonia was a common cause of death among the older people, but certainly the most prevalent disease was malaria. Typhoid epidemics were very common. Every community had typhoid fever every fall."

The nation was undergoing expansion. It was a period of great unrest. The industrial revolution began about 1820 and the movement from the farms to the cities was initiated. We were a nation of young people and the period was one of great vitality. The birth rate was high, how high we can only estimate, for there were no accurate records. A high death rate was almost inevitable.

In retrospect, it becomes quite clear that the prevalence of the great epidemics and, in fact, the very high over-all death rate, was not due to false epidemiological theories of physicians, nor lack of understanding of causal factors in illness. Rather, the epidemics were due, in great part, to social and economic factors that dominated the lives of all the people. Chief of these were:

1. Rapid rate of growth of the population due to the high birth rate and heavy immigration.

2. The industrialization of the eastern seaboard, with rapid increase in municipal population, and resulting overcrowding, bad housing, inadequate sanitary facilities, polluted municipal water supplies, contaminated food, myriads of flies and general prevalence of filth.

3. Rapid expansion of the West, with continuous movement of population. In fifty short years the nation extended from the Appalachian Mountains to the Pacific, and from the Canadian border to the Gulf of Mexico.

We were a virile, dynamic, exuberant, careless, restless pioneer people, with little regard for security or for human safety, willing to do or die, and many died. But life was cheap. Recklessness was a virtue. Every young man was anxious for adventure, willing to take his chances of survival, and to risk the hazards. The risks were great but the rewards of individual initiative were enormous. The watchword was: "Each man for himself. The devil take the hind-most," and the devil in the form of cholera, typhoid fever, and yellow fever often took the strongest, and the best as well.

Urbanization of the nation without proper understanding of the problems and hazards of crowded community life was one of the most important factors in the high death rate. The people utilized the same type of sanitary facilities and followed the same habits and customs that had been the common customs in the sparsely settled rural homes from which they had come. The results were disastrous.

Stephen Smith, in 1865, clearly understood the relationship of sickness to poverty, overcrowding, and bad social conditions. He says, "And when we remember that the great excess of mortality and of sickness in our city occurs among the poorer classes, and that such excessive unhealthiness and mortality is a public source of physical and social want, demoralization and pauperism, the subject of needed sanitary reforms in this crowded metropolis assumes such vast magnitude as to demand the most serious consideration of those who have regard for the welfare of their fellow beings, and the interests of their community."[12]

Bolduan, in his essay on *Public Health in New York City,* says, "New York appears to have been a reasonably clean and tidy town during the first quarter of the nineteenth century. The general death rate was about 25 per thousand, and the infant mortality ranged between 120 and 140 per thousand live births.

"The second quarter brought profound changes. Population growth became accelerated. Factories multiplied, immigration from Europe increased rapidly, standards of living were lowered, the housing situation became acute and conditions became more and more unsanitary."[13]

Let us for a moment view a cross section of the population of the United States in the year 1850, as revealed by the United States Census reports of that year. The total population was just over 23 million, of whom 15 per cent were Negroes, 11 per cent of which were free and 89 per cent slaves. The occupations of this population are shown in Table I. Nearly half of the free male population over 15 years of age worked on farms. If we add the

Negro field workers, we have estimated that there were about three and one-half million, of a total of 6.5 million employed persons, working on farms. Industry occupied only 30 per cent of the total labor, and professions classified as "requiring an education" occupied only 4 per cent of the working population. The very small proportion of persons in government service is striking.

TABLE I

EMPLOYMENT OF FREE MALE POPULATION
OVER 15 YEARS OF AGE
1850 CENSUS

OCCUPATION	AMOUNT	RATE (%)
Agriculture*	2,400,583	45.1
Industry—e.g. commerce, trade manufacturing, mechanical arts	1,596,265	29.9
Common labor—not agriculture	993,620	18.7
Seaman and Navigation	116,341	2.2
Law, medicine, and divinity	94,515	1.8
Other occupations requiring an education	95,814	1.8
Government service	24,966	0.5
Total	5,322,104	100.0

*We have made an approximate estimate of an additional one million Negroes over 15 years of age, engaged in agriculture—giving a total of about 3.5 million agricultural workers in a total of 6.5 million.

We have compared the age distribution of the population in the 1850 census with a similar age distribution in 1940. (See Graph 6.) This graph is, perhaps, the key to the high rate of epidemic disease. Over 50 per cent of the population were under 20 years of age, less than 10 per cent were over 50 years.

We have no accurate data concerning migration, but the distribution of foreign born in our largest cities gives us some insight into the social problems of the day. (See Table II.) The great

TABLE II

NATIVITY OF POPULATION (FOUR LARGEST CITIES)*
U. S. 1850 CENSUS

CITY	TOTAL	FOREIGN BORN	IRISH	GERMAN
New York	513,485	235,783 (45%)	26%	11%
Philadelphia	408,045	121,699 (30%)	17%	5%
Baltimore	165,983	35,492 (21%)	7%	11%
Boston	135,625	46,677 (34%)	26%	1.3%

*No accurate summaries for nation as a whole.

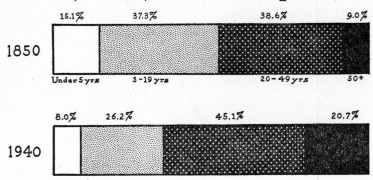

AGE DISTRIBUTION OF POPULATION IN THE UNITED STATES
1850 COMPARED WITH 1940

Per cent of Total Population in Each Age Group

	15.1%	37.3%	38.6%	9.0%
1850	Under 5 yrs	5 - 19 yrs	20 - 49 yrs	50+

	8.0%	26.2%	45.1%	20.7%
1940				

Data from U.S. Bureau of Census

Graph 6.—Comparison of the age distribution of population in the United States of 1850 with 1940. The shift to the left in this graph represents a major social change.

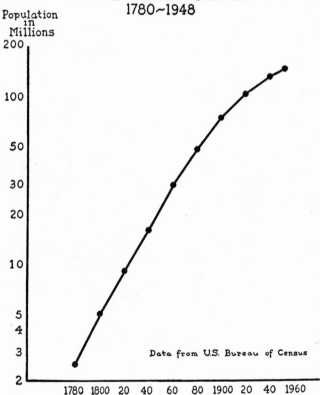

Graph 7.—The rate of growth of population in the United States (as indicated on a semilog scale) was most rapid during the early part of the nineteenth century.

proportion of immigrants were of German and Irish origin. The immigrants made up from one-third to one-half of the total population of New York, Philadelphia, Boston, and Baltimore.

The *rate* of growth of the nation is shown in Graph 7. It will be noted that the greatest rate of growth occurred during the first part of the nineteenth century. Graph 8 compares the *rate* of increase of rural and urban populations of the United States from 1800 to 1940. Urbanization began about 1820 and increased most rapidly during the first half of the century. Overnight, we became a nation of city-dwellers.

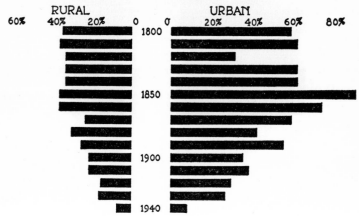

COMPARISON OF
INCREASE OF URBAN WITH RURAL POPULATION
IN THE UNITED STATES 1820~1940
PER CENT INCREASE OVER THE PREVIOUS CENSUS

Graph 8.—The rate of increase of urban as compared with rural population is an index of the industrialization of the nation. Our cities grew so rapidly that sanitary facilities could not keep pace.

A comparison of proportion of deaths by age group is given in Graph 9. We have compared Wiggleworth's famous table of 1789 with 1850, and 1850 with 1940. It will be seen that conditions were worse in 1850 than during the colonial period, with a particularly high fatality among children of school age.

There were over 300,000 deaths in 1850, and over 40 per cent of these deaths were due to "zymotic" diseases. These diseases took their heaviest toll in the younger age group, for in children of 5 to 9 years of age, 56 per cent of the deaths were from pestilential

EXPECTATION OF LIFE IN THE UNITED STATES
COMPARISON 1789 ~ 1850 ~ 1945

Proportion of Deaths by Age Groups in Total Mortality

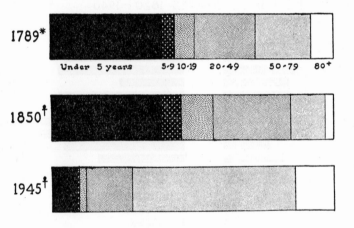

* Data from Wigglesworth's Table
‡ Data from United States Bureau of Census
Have made some interpolations because of difference in selected age groups

Graph 9.—The health situation in America was not improved but worsened during the first half of the nineteenth century. By 1945 the death rate in the age groups under 20 years had been reduced strikingly.

diseases. (See Table III.) We have no true measure of infant mortality, since there were no accurate records of birth, but we have some idea of the appalling death rate in infants from the ratio of infant deaths to total deaths. This ratio was 17 per cent in 1850 as compared with 7.4 per cent of total deaths in 1945.

TABLE III

DEATHS FROM ZYMOTIC DISEASES*

1850 CENSUS

Total deaths	323,023
Deaths from zymotic diseases	131,813
Per cent of deaths from zymotic diseases	40%

BY AGE GROUPS	
AGE GROUP	PER CENT OF TOTAL DEATHS FOR AGE GROUP
Children under 1 year	32
Children 1-4yrs. inclusive	54
Children 5-9 yrs. inclusive	56
Youths 10-19 yrs. inclusive	45
Adults 20-49 yrs. inclusive	39 (men 44—women 33)
Old age 50-79 inclusive	25

*Zymotic diseases do not include tuberculosis or pneumonia.

The deaths from zymotic diseases in 1850, by cause, are shown in Table IV. Cholera led the list that particular year, for it was a cholera year, but the deaths from other intestinal infections held a high rank. Table V gives a tabulation of all causes of death of infants; intestinal infections lead all the rest.

This analysis of the 1850 census gives us the answers to the questions we have asked at the outset of this discussion. Why was 1800 to 1870 the period of great epidemics? Why did these epidemics disappear and the crude death rate begin its steady decline before health services were organized, and before the advent of bacteriology with its knowledge of the cause of infection, and its incrimination of the individual patient as the important source of transmission of infectious diseases?

The data show that the great proportion of deaths were due to unfavorable environmental factors, to polluted water supplies, indescribable systems of feces disposal, overcrowding, with resultant disreputable housing conditions, bad milk, bad food, flies in millions, poor nutrition, long hours of overwork, and gross ignorance and carelessness.

TABLE IV

DEATHS FROM ZYMOTIC DISEASES
CENSUS OF MORTALITY 1850

DISEASE	TOTALS
1. Cholera	31,506
2. Dysentery and diarrhea	26,922
3. Fever—remittent, intermittent, intestinal	19,220
4. Typhoid fever	13,099
5. Croup (diphtheria)	10,706
6. Scarlet fever	9,584
7. Cholera infantum and cholera morbus	5,528
8. Whooping cough	5,280
9. Measles	2,983
10. Erysipelas	2,786
11. Smallpox	2,352

IMPORTANT INFECTIOUS DISEASES
NOT INCLUDED AS ZYMOTIC

Consumption (pulmonary tuberculosis)	33,516
Pneumonia (lobar)	12,130
Cephalitis—in children under 5 (chiefly cerebrospinal meningitis)	6,422
Convulsions and teething, chiefly in children under 2	6,072

TABLE V

INTESTINAL INFECTIONS OF INFANCY*
DEATHS IN CHILDREN UNDER 1 YEAR

DISEASE	TOTALS
Cholera infantum	1,111
Cholera morbus	908
Diarrhea	1,467
Dysentery	3,311
Cholera	1,417
Enteritis	645
Teething	836
Typhoid fever	391
Total	10,086
Total deaths in children under 1 yr.	54,265
Total deaths from zymotic diseases in children under 1 yr.	20,064

*Convulsions—2,844 deaths due in great part to intestinal infections, have been omitted.

The sanitary reform began about 1845. It was greatly aided by the Sanitary Conventions of 1857-1860. Although this reform was checked by the Civil War, it regained momentum at the end of the war, and by 1870 had a great impetus. The effects of these changes became apparent almost at once.

Our forefathers were quite wrong in their theories that disease was transmitted by miasmata, and, therefore, that community cleanliness was the only sure road to good health. The Sanitary Survey of New York City, by Stephen Smith and his associates, was concerned almost wholly with bad housing conditions, with no understanding of the actual causes of illness and death. But they concluded rightly that the "fever nests" of typhus, which they encountered, were due to the indescribably overcrowded, damp, dark basement housing of the recently arrived Irish immigrants, and that the enormous infant death rate of the summer months was a component part of poverty, ignorance, slums and filth.[14]

An awakening insight concerning those matters resulted in an aroused public consciousness. The newspapers, the church, businessmen, and the local sanitary services that were rapidly being formed, educated the people in the simple laws of community sanitation. Energetic efforts were undertaken to clean up the cities and to promote wholesome surroundings. "A clean city is a healthful city," was the slogan, and although it was only a part truth and based on faulty premises, nevertheless the results were most gratifying. Indeed, within a short period of time, the reduction of illness and death was really astounding.

Even malaria began to become circumscribed, not as a result of quinine, nor because of a knowledge that mosquitos transmitted the disease. The decline of malaria was a social phenomenon also. It was due to a transition from pioneer conditions to improved cultivation of the land, better rural housing, more cattle, more drainage of the bottom land, rapid transportation, replacement of the village mill and its mill pond by centralized milling, and all the other components of an advancing civilization.

The period of the great pestilences was on the wane; the period of exact bacteriological and epidemiological knowledge was about to dawn. Important as this new epoch was to be in saving life and preventing suffering, nevertheless, the most important factor of the whole century in reduction of illness and death was an awakening of a social consciousness in the nation. A development of compassion for the suffering of the poor, an aroused sense of public decency, a finer feeling for the value of human life; these resulted in the development of a sanitary consciousness, and this in turn resulted in the adoption and establishment of the simple principles of family and community cleanliness.

In truth, it was common sense, down-to-earth good community housekeeping, which led the way out of the wilderness of disease and disaster. The period of great epidemics was over.

SUMMARY

Community invasion by epidemic disease is an irresistible force which inspired the initiation of improved health services, and the promotion of general social betterment. Thus, the great epidemics of the 19th century in America were of paramount importance because of the impetus they gave to the initiation and consummation of sound health services for the nation.

An epidemic is an unexpected and very dramatic deviation from the normal. We have all observed the striking social phenomenon that any abrupt upheaval, any rapid and sharp deviation from the accustomed state of affairs, may arouse the people with an astounding force, amounting sometimes to an unreasoning panic.

The existing normal conditions may represent a very bad situation, for normal does not mean optimum, nor, in fact, does it mean even satisfactory conditions. A normal situation is, simply, one to which the individual, or the community, is accustomed, and to which it is adjusted.

The unhappy situation, in which the American people found themselves from 1800 to 1850, had become acceptable to them. It was recognized, of course, that the unsanitary living conditions, the gross overcrowding in cities, the poverty and ignorance of great masses of people contributed to the high morbidity, the appalling mortality in childhood and to the over-all high death rate. But these matters were regarded with equanimity as burdens to be borne, for they were omnipresent, of everyday occurrence, and certainly of no direct concern to government—local, state, or national.

But the epidemics, though comparatively infrequent, and relatively unimportant as causes of illness and death, were regarded as terrifying disasters, for the reason that they appeared so insidiously, so suddenly and struck with such dramatic force. As a result, immediate and vigorous action was taken to improve the whole sanitary situation. Thus we learn that it is the sudden and rapid deviation from the normal in our social or economic system, that first causes consternation of the people, and then serves as the catalyst in bringing about extensive social reforms.

References

1. Caulfield, E.: The Throat Distemper—1735-1740, Yale Journal of Biology and Medicine, 1939.
2. Rush, Benjamin: Medical Inquiries and Observations, Philadelphia, Vol. III, 4th ed., 1815.
3. Webster, Noah: A Brief History of Epidemic and Pestilential Diseases, Hartford, 1799, 2 vols.
4. Clot-Bey, Le Dr.: Sur la Peste, Paris, 1854.
5. Act for Making Provision for the Effective Performance of Quarantine, London, 1825.
6. Proceedings of the Third National Quarantine and Sanitary Convention, New York, 1859.
7. Jones, Joseph: Contagious and Infectious Diseases, Vol. I, Part I, p. 535, 1887.
8. Shattuck, Lemuel: The Report of the Sanitary Commission of Massachusetts, Boston, 1850.
9. Boyd, Mark: A Historical Sketch of the Prevalence of Malaria in North America, American Journal of Tropical Medicine 21: 223, 1941.
10. Reports of the New York City Sanitary Association, Academy of Medicine, 1859.
11. Dick, Everret: Professor of History, Union College, Nebraska, The Sod House Frontier, 1854-1890.
12. Report on the Sanitary Condition of New York City, Citizens Association, New York, 1865.
13. Bolduan, C. F.: The Public Health of New York City, Bulletin of New York City Health Department, June, 1943.
14. Smith, Stephen, and Associates: Report of the Sanitary Condition of the City of New York, 1865, D. Appleton and Co., N. Y.

III. THE BACTERIOLOGICAL ERA (1876-1920)

JAMES A. DOULL, M.D., DR.P.H., F.A.P.H.A.*

I. INTRODUCTION

IN SCIENCE, as in other fields of human endeavor, periods of great progress may be difficult to define precisely by the calendar. This is true of the Era of Bacteriology. Its beginnings were with ideas, some of which were ancient. It was immediately dependent upon discoveries in biology, chemistry, and physics, to which many minds contributed. Earlier clinical, pathological and epidemiological observations, moreover, had led a few outstanding thinkers to correct deductions regarding the origin of certain diseases. Such are the elements of a background covering a long period. It required the genius of Pasteur and of Koch to turn this background to account and to open a new chapter in human history.

The fundamental contribution was that of Pasteur who as early as 1862 published results of crucial experiments which ended the doctrine of spontaneous generation. If a single event may be selected as heralding the opening of the Bacteriological Era in epidemiology and medicine, the demonstration by Koch in 1876 of the essential role of a bacillus in anthrax is probably more significant than any other. General acceptance of the germ theory came quickly as other specific etiological agents were discovered or, lacking this, experimental proof of communicability was obtained. In arbitrarily choosing this date, it is essential to mention a few preceding and directly related events. In 1840 Henle laid down clearly the principles of the specific origin of infectious diseases; in 1844 Bassi demonstrated the association of a fungus with the muscardine disease of silkworms; in 1849 Pollender observed the bacillus of anthrax in animal tissues, as did Davaine in 1850, and in 1863 Davaine transferred anthrax by inoculation of healthy sheep with blood containing the minute rods, even when the blood was diluted a million times; in 1868 Villemin transmitted tuberculosis with tuberculous pus, and in 1874 Hansen showed that a bacillus was present in leprosy.

*Medical Director. Leonard Wood Memorial (American Leprosy Foundation).

Experimental proof of specificity of infectious diseases was an achievement of the greatest significance to medicine. It gave to epidemiology a secure foundation. Prior to this accomplishment, recognition and differentiation were dependent upon clinical signs and symptoms, supplemented latterly by gross and microscopical examinations of pathological tissues. Epidemiological theory, as Frost (1927) says, has since "been based firmly on a set of directly demonstrated facts which, in the earlier period, could only be inferred." Methods of isolation of microorganisms, together with discovery of a large number of other technical diagnostic aids, laid the basis for an extension of epidemiology on a scale previously impossible. Various forms of the principal diseases were identified and integrated, and, as physicians became familiar with laboratory tests and procedures, general recognition of infectious diseases and differentiation of infections producing similar clinical manifestations became accomplished facts.

The year 1920 is selected arbitrarily as marking the close of the Bacteriological Era. There is, however, some justification. The older methods of bacteriology had gradually become less productive and their failure to solve the riddle of the great influenza epidemic of 1918-1920 was conspicuous. By 1920 it had become clear that future progress depended chiefly on the development of new methods, especially for recognition and cultivation of the filtrable viruses.

Although known as the Bacteriological Era, great advances took place in other branches of biology, in chemistry, and in physics; and in the application of these basic sciences to medical problems. The rediscovery of Mendel's law opened new horizons in the study of hereditary factors. New diagnostic tools appeared, including the x-ray, the string galvanometer, the respiration calorimeter, among others, and several specific tests, including those of Widal, Wassermann, von Pirquet, and Schick. First antisepsis and then asepsis promoted the development of surgery. A new class of diseases, attributable to deficiency of specific elements in the diet, took its place in nosology. Beginnings were made in the differentiation of endocrine disorders. Medicine in general acquired an experimental basis, old concepts were discarded and a spirit of inquiry entered which permeated all its branches.

From a broader point of view, but likewise related to the development of epidemiology, the Era witnessed notable advances in almost all aspects of human affairs. When the period opened the telephone had just been invented; in 1896 the wireless telegraph was announced, and by 1920 radio communication was an established procedure. Advent of the automobile and the airplane revolutionized transportation. By the close of the period the use of electrical energy and the gas engine in industry, farming and domestic life had demonstrated that greater leisure and higher standards of living were potentially within the reach of all. Efforts to attain these goals are reflected in the tremendous strides in education and social organization which marked the period.

Current and Modern Concepts of Epidemiology.—Epidemiology, in the widest modern sense, deals with the study and interpretation of the mass phenomena of health and disease. Its unit is the population group rather than the individual. Its ideal methodology is the comparison of incidence rates for groups differing as far as is known only with respect to a single variable. Originally concerned only with epidemics, its scope was extended first to include infectious diseases which do not ordinarily occur in epidemic form, such as leprosy, syphilis, and tuberculosis, and later to noninfectious diseases, accidents, and certain normal physiological attributes for which group measurements can be obtained.

In so far as it may lay claim to be a science, epidemiology is collective, drawing its facts from the basic and medical sciences and from a large number of other sources, including sociology, demography and statistics, engineering, meteorology, and geography. These facts must be related in a consistent way to one another, to previous knowledge of a subject, and to biological phenomena in general. Their arrangement must permit the drawing of inferences, which may be limited, as, for example, citing the probable cause of a localized epidemic, or larger in scope, as explaining some peculiar phase of incidence, such as geographic, seasonal or age selection, or developing a theory applicable to the occurrence of epidemics in general.

During the Bacteriological Era the concept of epidemiology as a science was limited to the infectious diseases and it is with this particular group, and especially with the development of epidemiological theory relating to their occurrence and spread, that this review is chiefly concerned. The epidemiology of infectious diseases differs from that of other diseases and conditions in that it has a foundation of coherent and related facts. These concern the nature of infectious agents and the conditions which limit their reproduction and survival; the modes by which their transmission is effected and the type of clinical and immunological responses which they evoke, and the occurrence and frequency of reservoirs of infection in animals and of overt and concealed infections in man. The mass phenomena of infectious diseases thus have a common philosophy and are explained in accordance with these facts and in terms of exposure or dosage, susceptibility or its antithesis resistance, and variation in invasiveness and pathogenicity of living agents. This homogeneity distinguishes the infectious diseases and warrants a separate compartment for their epidemiology. Logically, this compartment should be extended to include not only the infectious diseases of man but also those of animals and of plants.

The modern extension of the subject matter of epidemiology has many advantages and any loss which epidemiology suffers in coherency and homogeneity is more than compensated for by a widening of knowledge through application of epidemiological methods to noninfectious diseases and other conditions. Strictly speaking, such application is of course not new, going back at least to Baker's study of the Devonshire Colic in the latter part of the eighteenth century. August Hirsch saw "the germ of a science" in the historical and geographic pathology of all afflictions of mankind. During the period under review there were many studies which today would be classed as epidemiological although the workers did not regard themselves as laborers in that field. These may be regarded as marking the transition of epidemiology from the infectious diseases to a wider sphere.

Even with the limited definition of epidemiology which prevailed, a reviewer of the period faces a difficult task. To obtain a comprehensive picture, it is necessary to consider progress made in a large number of fields. This could be done in detail only by a group of specialists. In selecting events for mention, therefore, serious errors of omission doubtless have been committed. A brief sketch is given of the matrix in which epidemiology grew, of epidemics, of American contributions to etiology, and of important extensions to epidemiological theory. A few examples are taken from field studies to illustrate the practical approach taken by American workers. There are included also three examples, from the last decade of the period, of epidemiological methods as applied to noninfectious conditions. An effort has been made throughout to avoid parochialism by placing American work in its proper perspective.

II. RELATED PROGRESS IN THE UNITED STATES

A review of the growth of epidemiology requires brief mention of progress in related fields which permitted its development.

Public Health Organization.—For the successful development of epidemiology, machinery for notification of morbidity and mortality must be set up. Well-organized health departments are essential. Health departments in turn are a product of maturing political organization. In 1876 there were in the Union 38 states, nine territories, the District of Columbia, and the unorganized territory of Oklahoma, with a total population of less than fifty millions. By 1920 all the territories had become states and the total population had increased to more than one hundred and five millions. In 1876 only eight states had health departments; in 1920 all states had health officers and many had large and well-staffed departments. City and county health work likewise progressed. There were no county health departments until 1908; in 1920 there were 131. Several of the larger cities entered the period with permanent boards of health; in 1920 nearly all had well-developed health departments. The first public health laboratory, a peculiarly American institution, was established by the city of New York in 1892. In 1908, that city also established the first Bureau of Child Hygiene, under the leadership of Josephine Baker. The Minnesota Board of Health was the first to appoint an epidemiologist; H. W. Hill was so designated in 1909 and a Division of Epidemiology was established in 1910.

On the federal level, the Public Health Service acquired authority in 1893 to cooperate with state and local health departments to prevent spread of human diseases between the states. Investigations carried out under this authority, and especially those on typhoid fever by Lumsden and his associates, were a powerful influence in the establishment of county health units, as was also the hookworm work of the Rockefeller Sanitary Commission and the Rockefeller Foundation. The laboratories now known as the National Institutes of Health were established in 1902, under an Act which directed the Service to undertake research into diseases of mankind and matters pertaining to public health. The Children's Bureau was established in 1912 and requires mention here especially because of its studies on infant mortality. Other bureaus of the Department of Labor were engaged in collection of social statistics and in research activities which were of fundamental importance; studies on fatigue and hours of labor and on the health of women in industry may be cited in particular. A complete review of epidemiology would require also discussion of some of the work of the Division (later Bureau) of Entomology established in the Department of Agriculture in 1878, the Bureau of Animal Industry established in 1884, the Weather Bureau (Department of Commerce) established in 1890, and the Bureau of Mines (Department of the Interior) established in 1910. One notable study from the Bureau of Animal Industry, that of Smith and Kilborne on Texas Fever of cattle, is discussed below. Reference will be made also to joint studies on industrial hygiene by the Bureau of Mines and the Public Health Service.

Demography and Vital Statistics.—The Bacteriological Era is likewise the Statistical Era and vital statistics are basic tools of the epidemiologist. Population studies of the Bureau of the Census became increasingly valuable with each decennial census. Registration systems for births and deaths were first established in a few of the larger cities. The reports for the state of Massachusetts go back to 1857. The federal Registration Area for Deaths was established in 1880, but at the beginning included only Massachusetts, New Jersey, District of Columbia, and a number of registration cities, altogether about 17 per cent of the population of the United States. In 1900 the federal government began to issue annual reports for the Registration Area. Reporting of smallpox, cholera, diphtheria, scarlet fever, or any other diseases dangerous to the public health was made compulsory by the Michigan State Board of Health in 1883 and according to Collins (1946) that state was the first to put reporting on a working basis. Massachusetts, which had a voluntary plan as early as 1876, made reporting compulsory in 1884.

Mention may be made here of certain outstanding American pioneers in vital statistics. In the early part of the period the outstanding figure was John Shaw Billings. A little later George C. Whipple, a sanitary engineer and teacher, developed the subject.

Still later refinements in statistical technics were introduced, notably by Raymond Pearl, a biologist and pupil of Karl Pearson.

One of the basic handicaps to the extension of epidemiology is the lack of current data on illnesses other than the infectious diseases and on the physical status of the population in general. According to Collins, the earliest tabulated morbidity data seem to be those of the English Friendly Societies which go back to the 1830's. The first attempts to collect general morbidity data in the United States were made at the time of the federal censuses of 1880 and 1890. Tabulations were made by Billings to show the prevalence of various illnesses on the day of the census. The first attempt to ascertain incidence was apparently a survey of slum dwellers in certain large cities, made in 1893 by the United States Department of Labor under the direction of Carroll D. Wright. These studies included questions about illnesses occurring within 12 months prior to the visit. In 1915-1917 Stecker, Frankel, and Dublin (1919) of the Metropolitan Life Insurance Company collected, through the agents of the company, a record of sickness among a half million policy holders. These surveys were scattered somewhat throughout the year and the duration of illness up to the time of the visit was obtained.

In searching for a sounder actuarial basis for health insurance, Warren and Sydenstricker (1916) of the Public Health Service reviewed available sources of statistics of disability, pointing out their scarcity and limitations. Unemployment on account of disability among members of representative local unions in Massachusetts and New York was studied and comparisons made with the records of the United States Army.

The medical examinations of drafted men in World War I provided, for the first time, statistics of prevalence of defects and diseases on a nation-wide basis, although restricted to males aged 18 to 30 years. The total number of men registered was approximately 10,000,000. Love and Davenport (1920) in an analysis of the records of 2,510,791 men found that by far the commonest defect was one or another type of deformity of the foot, sufficiently severe in 2 per cent of men examined to cause rejection. Hernia and enlargement of the inguinal rings constituted the second largest group. Then came in sequence, organic diseases and defects of the heart, defective vision and blindness, and defective physical development. Methods of detection were inadequate, but 55,631 cases (2.2 per cent) of frank tuberculosis of the lungs were diagnosed. In studying the frequency of these and of a large number of other conditions, the country was divided into 156 sections according to outstanding racial and occupational characteristics, and into urban and rural districts. Apart from its military and social significance the report is an encyclopedia of epidemiological information.

The first community survey for tuberculosis was conducted in 1917-1923 at Framingham, Massachusetts, by the National Tuberculosis Association with the financial support of the Metropolitan Life Insurance Company. A ratio of nine active cases to each annual death was estimated.

Two new and major sources of data on illness and disability were tapped during the period. These were school children and industrial workers.

Medical examination of school children began in France. Rosenau in his textbook *Preventive Medicine and Hygiene* (Sixth Edition) gives a review of developments in the United States. The first systematic inspection of school children was begun in Boston in 1894 by Samuel H. Durgin, Commissioner of Health. Prior to this, however, in 1890, Henry P. Bowditch had made an extensive and scientific examination of groups of school children, reported in an essay entitled: *The Growth of Children Studied by Galton's Method of Percentile Grades*. In 1908 there were 70 cities outside of Massachusetts which had medical inspection of schools. By 1924, 31 states and territories had enacted school inspection laws.

Availability of school children for examination was utilized early in studies of prevalence of various defects, goiter, and infectious diseases. For example, McMullen, Taliaferro Clark and others of the Public Health Service examined large numbers of school children in their investigations of trachoma in Kentucky, Virginia, West Virginia, and a few other areas. Sufficient house-to-house examinations of adults were made to establish the fact that the ratios for school children indicated fairly closely the relative levels of prevalence in the general population. In certain schools more than one sixth of the children were affected and in more than 5 per cent of the cases there was marked visual damage. A curious feature established in these studies is the relative immunity of the Negro to trachoma.

Industrial hygiene had its origins in England and Germany. Deaths by occupations for the Registration Area were published by the Bureau of the Census in 1890, 1900, 1908, and 1909, for general classes and for a few distinctive occupations. Proportional mortality studies gave some indication of the relative risks of certain occupations. Notable contributions relating to industrial hygiene and occupational hazards were made during the period by pioneers including Andrews, Frankel, Gorgas, Alice Hamilton, Hanson, Hayhurst, Hoffman, Kober, Lanza, Lee, Price, Sayres, Schereschewsky, G. W. Thomson, and others. In 1911, six states, California, Connecticut, Illinois, Michigan, New York, and Wisconsin, enacted laws requiring the reporting of certain occupational diseases.

At the suggestion of the National Tuberculosis Association, joint studies of conditions in the mines were undertaken by the Bureau of Mines and the Public Health Service soon after the establishment of the Bureau, and these agencies in 1914 also began an extensive series of investigations of dusty trades in general. The report by Lanza et al. (1917) of the prevalence of "Miners' Consumption" among zinc miners of southwestern Missouri, with x-ray studies of 150 patients, disclosed one of many serious situations which had been overlooked or neglected. Of 720 miners examined, 433 were affected, 103 having tubercle bacilli in their sputum. The examined persons represented only about one quarter of the hard rock miners of the district and if it be assumed that all those not examined were free from the disease, which could not have been the case, the prevalence rate would still be 15 per cent. The authors considered that the true figure was between 30 and 35 per cent.

An extensive study was made of the health and physical status of workers in the garment industry by Schereschewsky and Tuck (1915). No vocational disease was discovered. The study, however, has many interesting points. The complexity of occupational studies was clearly demonstrated by the fact that among 722 pressers there were represented 77 previous occupations. A very large number of physical defects was noted, an average of more than four per individual. The prevalence rate of tuberculosis was for females three times and for males ten times the prevalence among soldiers of the United States Army, but a tendency of persons with tuberculosis to turn to a sedentary occupation and poor environmental conditions of the garment workers outside the factory were probably important factors. The commoner defects which were discovered were defective vision (69 per cent); faulty posture (50 per cent); chronic nose and throat affections (26.2 per cent); defective teeth (26.0 per cent), and defective hearing (10 per cent).

Progress in Professional Education.—Manifestly, well-trained physicians and public health officers are essential for the development of epidemiology. In 1876, when William H. Welch made his first trip to Europe, teaching laboratories were unknown in American medical schools. Medical education made enormous strides especially following the Abraham Flexner report in 1910.

Beginnings were made in the education of health officers. In January, 1889, the first special laboratory in America devoted to teaching and research in hygiene was opened at the University of Michigan under the direction of Victor C. Vaughan. Vaughan was a bacteriologist of broad experience and vision, and a great teacher of epidemiology and public health. His chair at Michigan included both hygiene and physiological chemistry and he developed methods for studying the chemical composition of bacteria. He was a member of the commission which studied the sanitary conditions in United States Army camps during the Spanish-American War. In 1891, Alexander C. Abbott, a pupil and colleague of Welch, went to the University of Pennsylvania to develop a hygienic laboratory established a short time before by Billings. At the Massachusetts Institute of Technology, courses for health officers were introduced by William T. Sedgwick, a great teacher and investigator whose influence on sanitary science and public health was tremendous. In these institutions chief emphasis was quite naturally placed on bacteriology and on the infectious diseases, as was the case in Great Britain and in Germany. The School of Hygiene and Public Health at Johns Hopkins University, established in 1916, was the first institution to include in its curriculum all major disciplines which contribute to public health in its broader aspects and to provide a faculty competent in these fields. There the first university department of epidemiology was organized with Wade H. Frost as Resident Lecturer and later as Professor. The funds for this school were provided by the Rockefeller Foundation after study and recommendations were made by

Wickliffe Rose and William H. Welch, and Welch and W. H. Howell were responsible for its organization and early development.

Two other pioneers should be mentioned. George M. Sternberg was a notable bacteriologist and administrator. As Surgeon General of the Army, he appointed the Yellow Fever Commission, was instrumental in the establishment of the Army Medical School, and guided a generation of military hygienists.

George M. Kober was a medical teacher and hygienist whose broad interests included industrial health and social betterment. As a professor at Georgetown Medical School from 1889 he took an active interest in the sanitation of the District of Columbia, calling attention to the undue prevalence of typhoid as early as 1890.

III. EPIDEMICS

The direction of epidemiological investigation during the period naturally was determined largely by occurrence of epidemics. Reference will be made later to specific contributions but it is necessary at this point to give some account of certain epidemics which destroyed large numbers of persons and seriously disrupted normal community organization and activities.

Yellow Fever.—Yellow fever had long been a scourge of the tropics and had been introduced repeatedly into American ports. In 1878, an epidemic occurred which ultimately spread to eight states but was seen in its greatest intensity in Memphis, Tennessee. The pre-epidemic population of that city was about 50,000. Of these, about 30,000 fled. In a space of three months, 17,500 of the remainder were attacked and 5,150 died. Of a police force of 48 officers, 27 were attacked and 10 died. Of 39 members of the Howard Association who volunteered to stay and assist the sick, 32 were attacked and 12 died. Such was yellow fever when it struck a large and susceptible population. The last epidemics in the United States occurred in 1905 at Galveston and New Orleans.

Influenza.—Pandemic influenza occurred in 1889-1890 and again in 1918. Only isolated facts are known regarding the beginnings of the 1889 pandemic. Forty years had intervened since the pandemic of 1847-1848 and few living physicians had had any experience with it. At first it was thought to have originated in Siberia (Russian Influenza) in May, 1889, but later it was reported to have been prevalent in western Canada at about the same time. In the summer of 1889, a severe type was reported in Greenland and in October it was recognized in England. On December 17, it was reported in New York City and within 10 days there were hundreds of cases. By the end of December, it was prevalent in nearly all large cities of the east and middle sections and within three months from first recognition it had literally covered the country. The mortality rate from respiratory diseases, and from all causes, was everywhere increased. In the Twenty-First Annual Report of the State Board of Health for Massachusetts, Abbott states that the duration of the epidemic in that state was about seven weeks and estimated that 850,000 persons, or 40 per cent, of the population of the state were attacked. An estimate of 20 to 30 per cent for England was made by Parsons. A second wave occurred in the United States in March and April, 1891, and in England at the same time, but a large part of Europe escaped this phase. A third wave occurred in England in October of the same year and in the United States in December. A recurrence of this wave in January, 1892, was more severe in the United States than the original outbreak of 1889.

Localized outbreaks of influenza occurred in many parts of the country between 1892 and 1910. Between 1910 and 1915 there is no evidence of any epidemic, mortality rates from influenza and pneumonia being exceptionally regular throughout the United States Registration Area for Deaths. In December, 1915, and in January, 1916, a sharp rise in mortality from respiratory diseases occurred which was almost universal and synchronous throughout the United States. In the Public Health Reports for January 7, 1916, influenza was reported to be epidemic in 23 states, a fact now generally forgotten.

Outbreaks of an influenza-like disease occurred in certain army camps in the United States in March, 1918, and even earlier the presence of influenza was reported from certain ships and stations of the United States Navy. At about the same time or a little later "three day fever" was prevalent in armies on the Western European Front. In June, influenza was recognized to be prevalent in Continental Europe, England, and China. These spring and summer outbreaks have been called the first wave. In the United States the second wave or main epidemic broke explosively in October, being reported first from Boston. The third wave began in January, 1919, and continued through March. From studies of the United States Public Health Service to be mentioned later, about 22 per cent of inhabitants of 12 cities were attacked during the second wave and the case fatality varied from 0.8 to 3.1 per cent. The pandemic caused an increase in the general death rate for 1918 of the Continental United States of more than three per 1,000; that is, it caused an excess of at least 300,000 deaths. That is what would be expected if there had been 20,000,000 persons attacked (about 20 per cent of the population) and the average case fatality rate had been 1.5 per cent. The epidemic, however, extended into 1919, and a study by Collins, Frost, Gover, and Sydenstricker (1930) showed that in 35 large cities with a population of about 20 millions the excess mortality for the epidemic period of 31 weeks was 550 per 100,000; that is, about 110,000 deaths. For the whole country, therefore, the mortality caused by the epidemic may have been about a half million deaths, more or less.

Typhoid Fever.—Records of outbreaks of gastrointestinal diseases constitute a black chapter in the nation's sanitary history. During the Spanish-American War, Reed, Vaughan, and Shakespeare (1904) reported that about one fifth of soldiers in national encampments in the United States contracted typhoid fever. During 1900 in the United States there were about 35,000 deaths from typhoid and paratyphoid fevers. This would indicate that there were at least 350,000 cases and probably nearly twice as many in a population of 76,000,000, or that at least one person in 217 was attacked and perhaps one in 109. During the 40 years from 1880 to 1920 it can be stated conservatively that *more than a million persons* died from typhoid and paratyphoid fevers in the United States. Water, milk, and shellfish contributed their quota of epidemics, especially in large cities, but in the country as a whole the bulk was autumnal typhoid, caused principally by contamination of food directly by typhoid carriers or indirectly through the medium of flies.

Diphtheria and Scarlet Fever.—When the period opened, very high mortality rates prevailed from scarlet fever and diphtheria, violent and severe outbreaks being very common. In New York City in 1881 more than one per cent of children under 10 years of age died from diphtheria; in 1920 not one in a thousand died from the disease. For the Registration States of 1900 the death rate from diphtheria and croup was 40.4 per 100,000 in 1900; 22.5 in

1910 and 17.3 in 1920. For scarlet fever the comparable rates were 9.6 in 1900; 12.2 in 1910, and 5.2 in 1920. Only a very few epidemics of these diseases were attributed to contamination of milk or milk products.

Anterior Poliomyelitis.—An epidemic of anterior poliomyelitis occurred in Rutland, Vermont, in 1894, the first to be described in the United States. The first large epidemic occurred in and around New York City in 1907. During the years 1907 to 1910, epidemics occurred in Massachusetts, Minnesota, Iowa, and New York. From 1910 on, poliomyelitis became more frequent and widespread, culminating with the great epidemic of 1916 which caused at least 29,000 cases and 6,000 deaths.

Miscellaneous Outbreaks.—In 1898-1899 cerebrospinal meningitis was reported in 27 states, but in a mild form. In 1904-1905 a very serious outbreak occurred in New York City. In 1911 there were cases in several southern states and in 1912 there was a severe epidemic in Texas. It was a serious problem also in certain Army camps during World War I. Smallpox was continually present in one or another part of the country, but epidemics were limited by vaccination campaigns. The fatality rates varied greatly from as low as 0.3 per cent to as high as 25 per cent. Mild and severe epidemics, respectively, seemed to remain true to type giving rise to the opinion that two different strains prevailed. After 1900, with a few exceptions, all outbreaks were of the mild form. For the Registration States of 1900 the death rate was 0.3 per 100,000 in 1900; 0.5 in 1910, and 0.1 in 1920. Plague was first reported in 1900 at San Francisco. Numerous outbreaks of botulism occurred between 1899 and 1920, especially in California. In 1911 a small outbreak of brucellosis was described in southwest Texas which is of particular significance in that it was the first outbreak attributable to goat's milk to be described in the United States. Encephalitis lethargica (nona) was noted in 21 states in 1918 and 1919.

IV. AMERICAN CONTRIBUTIONS TO ETIOLOGY

The majority of early discoveries in microbiology were made by Europeans, trained in the methods of Pasteur and Koch. Americans, nevertheless, made important contributions, of which the following is by no means a complete list: the first to describe and present adequate proof of the specific relationship of a micro-organism to disease was Theobald Smith (1889), who discovered *Babesia (Piroplasma) bigemina* in the red blood cells of cattle suffering from Texas fever; Welch and Nuttall (1892) described *Clostridium welchii,* the principal cause of gas gangrene in man; Theobald Smith (1896) differentiated between human and bovine types of *Mycobacterium tuberculosis;* Flexner (1900) described an important member of the Shigella group; Howard and Perkins (1901) described *Streptococcus mucosus* (probably *Pneumococcus,* Type III); Stiles (1902) recognized that the species of hookworm prevailing in this country was a new one, *Necator americanus;* Carlisle (1906), Norris, Pappenheimer, and Flournoy (1906), and Novy and Knapp (1906) described *Borrelia novyi,* which causes American relapsing fever, and Noguchi (1912) cultivated this microorganism; Ricketts (1906a) transmitted Rocky Mountain spotted fever to guinea pigs and monkeys; Ricketts (1909) and Wolbach (1919) described *Rickettsia rickettsii,* which causes Rocky Mountain spotted fever; Anderson and Goldberger (1912) demonstrated the identity of Brill's disease and Mexican typhus (tabardillo); Ferry (1911) described *Hemophilus bronchisepticus,* a rare parasite of man but a frequent cause of bronchopneumonia in rodents; McCoy and Chapin (1912) isolated *Pasteurella tularensis* from ground squirrels, Wherry and Lamb (1914) the same microorganism from a human case of ulcerative conjunctivitis and Wherry (1914) from wild rabbits, and Francis (1919) identified it as the cause of Deerfly fever of Utah; Strong and associates (1915) described in detail a microorganism found in various tissues in Oroya fever, presumably the same as that previously observed by Barton in red blood cells, and named it *Bartonella bacilliformis;* and Evans (1918) made an important contribution by discovering affinity between *Brucella melitensis* and *Brucella abortus.*

Reed, Carroll, Agramonte, and Lazear (1900) reported transmission of yellow fever to human subjects, to which reference will be made later. Reed and Carroll (1902) showed that the virus of yellow fever is filtrable; Hektoen (1905) transmitted measles to human beings, and Anderson and Goldberger (1911) the same disease to monkeys; Ashburn and Craig (1907) showed that the causal agent of dengue fever is filtrable, and Flexner and Lewis (1909) confirmed observations of Landsteiner and Popper (1909) on susceptibility of monkeys to anterior poliomyelitis and first accomplished transmission with filtrates. Rous (1910; 1911) described a transplantable tumor of fowls and later he and his associates two other tumors, all transmissible from diseased to healthy fowls by inoculation of cell-free Berkefeld filtrates. These findings, although having no known relationship to tumors of man, gave great impetus to experimental studies of virus diseases of man and animals. There should also be mentioned cultivation by Harrison (1906-1907) of tissue cells *in vitro*, the basis for modern methods of virus cultivation.

Two outstanding clinical contributions to etiology of infectious diseases should be included. Koplik (1896) described characteristic spots on the buccal mucous membrane, "absolutely pathognomonic of beginning measles," and Brill (1898) described a mild febrile disease resembling typhoid fever but without the Widal reaction, later recognized as typhus, occurring in New York City.

V. IMPORTANT EPIDEMIOLOGICAL PRINCIPLES ESTABLISHED

During the period two great extensions of knowledge took place which were of fundamental importance to epidemiology. These were (1) transmission by arthropods, in some instances from an animal reservoir, and (2) transmission by healthy carriers. Prior to establishment of these principles, the clinical case was regarded as the sole source of infection and the chief control measures were strict isolation of the patient and disinfection of clothing and other articles presumed to have been contaminated by him. To explain lack of association between cases, particles of infectious material were assumed to be spread by air currents or carried distances on persons and objects, and to convey infection after months or even years.

1. **Transmission by Arthropods.**—Manson (1878) had observed metamorphosis of the microfilaria of *Filaria bancrofti* in Culex mosquitoes but the first proof of transmission by arthropods came from the experiments of Theobald Smith and Kilborne (1893), who showed not only that Texas fever of cattle is transmitted by a tick *(Boöphilus annulatus),* but the even more remarkable fact that the infection is transmitted by the progeny of ticks which mature on infected cattle. Malaria was the first human disease for which complete proof of arthropod transmission was obtained and

chief credit goes to European investigators, except for a fundamental observation of fertilization in *Halteridium,* a parasite of birds, by W. G. MacCallum. At the Twenty-Eighth Annual Meeting of The American Public Health Association, Reed, Carroll, Agramonte, and Lazear (1900) presented a preliminary report of their classic experimental work on the transmission of yellow fever from man to man by *Aëdes egypti.*

King (1906) and Ricketts (1906b) independently showed that Rocky Mountain spotted fever in guinea pigs could be transmitted by the wood tick *(Dermacentor andersoni),* and Ricketts (1907a, b) demonstrated that ticks were naturally infected and that the infected female may transmit the infection to the next generation through her eggs. Between 1896 and 1903 several foreign investigators had shown that plague was primarily a disease of rats transmitted by fleas and this was confirmed by the English Plague Commission (Report of 1906). In 1903 Rupert Blue suspected that the ground squirrel in California had become infected, and five years later natural infection of these rodents was demonstrated by McCoy (1908) and by Wherry (1908). Credit should be given here to a Brazilian scientist, Carlos Chagas (1909), for experimental transmission of South American trypanosomiasis by the infected *Triatoma megista.* In 1916 British workers transmitted trench fever to healthy persons by inoculation of blood from patients; transmission by body lice which had fed on febrile patients was accomplished by the Medical Research Commission of the American Red Cross (Report, 1918).

2. **Carriers.**—Sternberg (1880-1881) had found a diplococcus resembling that causing pneumonia in the saliva of a well person and Loeffler (1884) isolated *Corynebacterium diphtheriae* from a healthy throat. The importance of carriers as sources was, however, first emphasized by Koch (1893) in studies of cholera. Healthy carriers of *Eberthella typhosa* were first demonstrated by Drigalski and Conradi (1902). Healthy carriers of *Neisseria meningitidis* were discovered by Albrecht and Ghon (1901) and another European, Glover (1920), demonstrated their epidemiological significance in 1915-1919. In the United States important contributions on prevalence of carriers were made by Park and Beebe (1894), who found 2.4 per cent of 330 healthy persons in New York City to be harboring virulent diphtheria bacilli; by Buerger (1905), who reported *Diplococcus pneumoniae* in 50 per

cent of normal mouths; by Rosenau, Lumsden, and Kastle (1909) who, in the first investigation of the general public for the purpose, found three typhoid carriers among 986 well persons in Washington, D. C.; by Anderson (1912), who reported that examination of 34,000 specimens of feces for the cholera vibrio at the New York Quarantine Station had revealed 28 positives in sick persons and 27 in well persons; by Flexner, Clark, and Fraser (1913), who demonstrated presence of virus of anterior poliomyelitis in healthy persons, and by Avery, Chickering, Cole, and Dochez (1917), who greatly extended and refined knowledge of pneumococcus carriers. Outbreaks of disease, especially typhoid fever, were frequently attributed to carriers during the period. The first instance to attract attention in the United States was that of "Typhoid Mary." The circumstances of the discovery of this carrier and the story of her career as a source of typhoid over a period of years have been described by G. A. Soper (1919), who discovered her in 1906.

VI. IMMUNITY FROM SUBCLINICAL INFECTION

The phenomenon of bacterial invasion without disease, symptomless and clinically unrecognizable, was called "sub-infection" by Adami (1899) with reference to the penetration of the colon bacillus into the portal blood stream. Brouardel and Thoinot (1905) applied the term "mithridatization" to the process of immunization of city dwellers to typhoid fever as a result of repeated minute doses of infection, insufficient to produce typhoid even in an abortive form. The reviewer is unaware of the origin of the term "subclinical infection." It was perhaps first used by Frost; certainly he more than any other popularized its use.

It was the study of diphtheria which brought greatest support to the theory of immunity from subclinical infection. Abel (1894) first detected antitoxin in blood of persons not known to have had diphtheria and we are indebted to him and other Europeans for basic knowledge of this subject. The Schick test made mass surveys possible and Park and Zingher (1914-1915) commenced studies in New York City which confirmed the relationship of age to acquirement of antitoxic immunity and demonstrated the positive association between immunity and aggregation of population. Carriers were demonstrated to be common and, from experimental evidence, it was assumed that active antitoxic immunity, naturally acquired, resulted only from specific infection.

Suggestive facts came also from the study of poliomyelitis. Lovett and Richardson (1911) from their studies in Massachusetts in 1907-1910 suggested that failure of poliomyelitis to visit the same district in successive years was an expression of immunity attained by the inhabitants. In Sweden, Wernstedt (1912) hypothecated a widespread diffusion of the virus as the most plausible explanation of the escape in 1911 of communities attacked in 1905. The younger average age of attack in cities than in rural areas, noted by Frost and mentioned below, is considered to be a result of earlier immunization in crowded communities.

The theory that immunizing infections are many times more frequent than are clinical attacks offers the most satisfactory explanation yet advanced for the age selection of diphtheria, scarlet fever, anterior poliomyelitis, and certain other diseases.

VII. ILLUSTRATIVE EXAMPLES OF EVOLUTION

The evolution of American epidemiology during the period may be illustrated further by examples from three classes of field investigations: (1) studies designed to extend knowledge of diseases in which the principal facts of their epidemiology had already been established, and (2) those of an exploratory nature in diseases of unknown etiology or in which established facts were meagre. In Class 1 there is frequently a background of information relating to the microorganism, which guides the investigator and adds weight to his conclusions. A third class is added to illustrate the profitable application of epidemiological methods to noninfectious conditions, an application which was to be greatly extended at a later date.

Class 1: Principal Facts Already Established

1. **Investigation of Epidemics of Typhoid Fever.**—Epidemics of typhoid fever in rapidly-growing American cities repeated the experience of Europe. Careful investigations made the mass characteristics of epidemics due to contaminated water or milk familiar to health officers. Concurrent laboratory studies laid the base for present bacteriological standards for drinking water, milk, and shellfish and it may be noted that the first attempt at standardization of procedures in water analysis was made by a committee

of the American Public Health Association in 1905. Many examples might be cited from the early investigations but a few will suffice.

The first outbreak of typhoid fever ascribed to pollution of drinking water was observed in North Boston, New York, in 1843 by Austin Flint (1845). The first large epidemic, definitely waterborne, to be recorded in the United States occurred at Plymouth, Pennsylvania, and was investigated by L. H. Taylor (1885). In a population of 8,000 persons there occurred 1,004 cases and 114 deaths within a few weeks. Plymouth received its water from a mountain stream which drained an *almost* uninhabited watershed. Nevertheless, the probable source was a man who lived in a house only 40 feet from the stream. He had contracted typhoid in Philadelphia in December, returned home well and relapsed, being still desperately ill on March 19. His dejecta were thrown on the bank of the stream but, because of freezing weather, could not have entered the water until a thaw occurred between March 25 and 31. The first case occurred on April 9. The users of well water, although in some instances living on the same streets as those who used the municipal supply, escaped.

In the winter of 1890-1891 typhoid epidemics occurred in Lawrence and Lowell, Massachusetts, that in Lowell being investigated by Sedgwick (1893). The major source of drinking water for both cities was the Merrimack River, the intake for Lawrence being nine miles nearer the sea than that for Lowell. The Lowell situation was complicated in that there were five water supplies, two of which were heavily polluted. By painstaking analysis of data on 550 cases, Sedgwick incriminated the principal municipal supply. He eliminated other possible vehicles and further supported his conclusion by discovering that, shortly before the outbreak, excreta from typhoid patients had been discharged into the river three miles above the intake. Lowell emptied its sewage into the Merrimack and an epidemic in Lawrence followed promptly. Later, Lawrence installed a slow sand filter and its "normal" winter typhoid was greatly reduced.

Hill (1911a) investigated very thoroughly a water-borne outbreak of typhoid which occurred at Mankato, Minnesota, in 1908. The season was unusual—June and July. There had been heavy rains between May 20 and June 24, causing a tremendous flood. Sewers were inadequate to take care of the water and sewage entered the wells supplying the town with drinking water. Great efforts were made to obtain complete registration of cases and the final figures showed 511 with 35 deaths, a fatality rate of 6.8 per cent, the rate being highest in children and those over 30 years of age. There was an unusual excess in females—219 cases in males and 292 in females. Hill noted also that 21 persons contracted the disease who had been visitors in the town for only one or two days and that the average incubation period in these cases was 13 $17/21$ days. The Mankato epidemic was preceded by 4,000 to 6,000 cases of diarrhea; that is, about one half of those drinking the water were affected. Extensive outbreaks of diarrhea preceding water-borne typhoid have been reported both in Europe and America and, while some or all may have been bacillary dysentery, their etiology is not known.

The first milk-borne outbreak of typhoid fever to be reported occurred at Penrith, England, in 1857, and was described by M. W. Taylor (1858). In 1895, Stamford, Connecticut, suffered a serious epidemic which was ably investigated by H. E. Smith (1896). The population numbered approximately 15,000. The epidemic began on April 14 and within nine days there were some 160 cases and 24 suspected cases. By the end of May there had occurred 386 cases. More than one third were in children less than ten years old. There were 125 houses with multiple cases in a total of 255 invaded. Ninety-five per cent of the cases were traced to the use of milk from one dairy which supplied 9 per cent of the total supply. At this dairy the milk cans were washed in water from a polluted well.

Conn (1895) described an outbreak of typhoid at Wesleyan University and for the first time showed conclusively the association of the disease with the eating of raw oysters. He used great care in eliminating other possible vehicles and supported his case by demonstrating that water in which the oysters had been placed for "fattening" had been polluted by sewage from a house in which typhoid recently had occurred.

A very large number of excellent descriptions of typhoid epidemics are to be found in the reports of state and city health departments and in the Public Health Reports, especially for the last decade of our period. For the earlier part, reference is made to Whipple (1908).

2. **Studies of Endemic Typhoid.**—Water-borne typhoid was relatively of much less importance in southern than in northern states.

In their studies of endemic typhoid fever in Richmond, Va., Levy and Freeman (1908) drew attention to the fact that the classic water-borne epidemics had all occurred in northern cities and most of them in other than the summer months. The usual peak in Richmond occurred in summer at which time the cases were pretty generally distributed over the city except that areas supplied by wells and without sewerage suffered most. A winter outbreak in January and February, 1908, showed an entirely different geographic picture, being almost entirely confined to the old city which was supplied with city water. An area supplied from a different intake than the larger supply had only a small proportion of the cases. The areas of the city spared in the summer months but supplied with city water suffered as heavily as the rest of the old city.

Reports of Rosenau, Lumsden, and Kastle and other workers of the Public Health Service (1907) on typhoid in the District of Columbia are notable in several respects. They were the first long-time studies of an endemic disease in the United States; they were comprehensive in that they included case investigations, sanitary engineering surveys, and bacteriological and chemical studies of water, ice, milk, and other foods; and they directed attention to the importance of insanitary conditions and contact in the spread of typhoid, especially in the warmer months. Actually, taking the country as a whole, these factors were very much more important than drinking water, milk, and shellfish in the transmission of typhoid fever, as was emphasized by Chapin.

3. **Epidemics of Dysentery.**—Water-borne outbreaks of dysentery were not commonly reported in the United States during the period. Hill (1911b) described four in Minnesota which were probably bacillary dysentery, although bacteriological evidence is lacking. In 1907, at Hibbing, about 2,000 persons were attacked in a population of 8,000. The cause apparently was pollution of a well by workmen making repairs. At St. Peter there were outbreaks in 1908 and 1909, both due to polluted river water entering a reservoir. At the University Agricultural College a deep well was contaminated by the backing up of a sewer and almost all who drank the water developed dysentery. The diarrhea which preceded the Mankato typhoid epidemic has already been mentioned.

4. **Septic Sore Throat.**—Milk-borne outbreaks of this disease had been described in England and the disease was considered to be caused by a streptococcus either of human or bovine origin.

The first large outbreak described in the United States occurred in Boston in 1911. This outbreak, which was investigated by Winslow (1912), was sharply explosive. A high proportion of the patients were users of milk from a dairy which furnished only a small percentage of the total supply. Multiple cases in families were common; there was an excess among females, and young adults were attacked more than children.

5. **Endemic Diphtheria and Scarlet Fever.**—The work of Chapin is well known to American students. He was the first systematically to collect equivalent data for patients and for members of their families. Frost (1938) has given an illuminating account of Chapin's use of these records in the measurement of infectiousness of diphtheria and scarlet fever by means of the secondary attack rate. After commenting on the fact that, although there was in the literature a tremendous mass of observations on the concentration of communicable diseases within the household, knowledge of the subject was diffuse and unorganized, partly because the observations were presented in a variety of forms not readily convertible to a common denominator, Frost says:

"The method which Dr. Chapin used for quantitative description of familial aggregation, a method which, so far as I have been able to ascertain, was introduced by him,* is the so-called 'secondary attack rate'; that is, the attack rate, within a specified time, in members of attacked families exclusive of the 'primary' case, time being reckoned from the onset of this case. The method itself is familiar; but before discussing its history it may be appropriate to call attention to its special merits—simplicity, and adaptability to a variety of uses."

The secondary attack rate answers directly the practical question of the risk to other members of the household within a specified period of time following occurrence of a case of communicable disease. It has also "broader significance in contributing to better understanding of the natural history of communicable diseases, especially the directly transmitted endemic infections for which the human host is obligatory. For such diseases the secondary attack rate gives the best approximation we have to the limits of incidence of the clinically recognized disease—or equally of the subclinical infection where it can be independently observed—in a group sub-

---

*"It is of course impossible to be certain that this method had not been used and presented in some earlier publication; but the evidence available to me indicates pretty clearly that Dr. Chapin devised the procedure to meet his own needs, and it is certain that its general use in this country derives from his work."

jected to almost certain physical exposure to the infective agent. More extended knowledge of these limits is of fundamental importance, not only for comparison of one disease with another, but equally for comparing the manifestations of the same disease in different areas and different periods of time."

In 1903 Chapin used the secondary attack rate in estimating the benefit to other members of the family of removal of a patient with diphtheria to the hospital. His report for 1908 gives secondary attack rates for scarlet fever and in this and subsequent reports he studied for that disease such questions as the benefit of removal to hospital, rates in families employing servants and nurses, and the rates in household associates with and without a history of previous attack.

6. Malaria.—Extensive field and laboratory investigations of malaria which increased greatly knowledge of the parasite, effective vectors, and methods of control, were carried out in the last decade of the period, especially by workers of the Public Health Service, including Carter, von Ezdorf, Griffitts, Mitzmain, Le Prince, Metz, and others whose publications are to be found chiefly in Public Health Reports from 1912 to 1920.

Class 2: Exploratory Studies

1. Yellow Fever.—The determination of the "extrinsic incubation period" of yellow fever by Henry R. Carter (1900) is an example both of brilliant deduction and of persistency in testing and retesting an hypothesis. Carter commenced his studies on the limits of incubation in 1887, having in mind a more satisfactory basis for quarantine measures. In 1898 at Orwood, Miss., he observed that intervals between the introduction of the first infecting cases and the occurrence of the first secondary cases varied from 11½ to 23 days. The time necessary to infect the environment was estimated from these and other observations to be from 10 to 17 days. The extraordinary accuracy of Carter's deductions is shown by the fact that Reed and his colleagues in their experimental work set the time required for maturation in the mosquito at 12 to 18 days.*

---

*Attention may be directed here to the similarity of these observations to those made by Smith and Kilborne (1893) in Texas fever of cattle. When susceptible cattle were exposed to infected animals on an uninfected field, the period lapsing before the disease developed was generally over 45 days and the first deaths occurred one to two weeks later. Cattle placed on an infected field sometimes died in less than 15 days after exposure. The explanation given was that ripe ticks falling from infected cattle laid their eggs in about seven days; these hatched in about 20 days and the newly-hatched young were at once ready to crawl on and infect cattle. The time of hatching varied with the temperature. The authors were unable to determine (p. 117) whether the tick is "a necessary or a merely accidental bearer of the microparasite."

Less well known are Carter's (1916-1917) observations on immunity conferred by an attack of yellow fever. At the time of his study the opinion was widely held that recurrent attacks of yellow fever were common. To quote:

"Obviously the natural method of testing this question is by observation of the exposure of men who have had yellow fever to the infection of that disease, and determining if they contract it again. The existence of the infection and degree of exposure would be judged of by the proportion of cases contracted by those who had *not* had yellow fever similarly exposed to infection-controls. If a negative result is reported, the observation would be convincing in proportion to the number of supposedly immune men thus exposed; the intervals from their last attacks; the degree of exposure, and the certainty that secondary attacks did not occur among men.

"Such observations are not rare, for instance at the end of 1879 there must have been a very small proportion of the population of New Orleans, Mobile, and the coast towns between them who had not suffered an attack of yellow fever in that or in previous years. They were free from yellow fever until 1897. In that year and 1898 there were widespread epidemics, yet recurrent attacks were reported in extremely few cases in these towns in 1897 and 1898— eighteen years later. Certainly no considerable number of well-marked cases could have occurred in those years. The same is true of many other epidemics and many other towns in the United States. We can readily present, then, a large number of people having had one attack of yellow fever exposed, after sufficiently long intervals, to infections very prevalent among those who had not had yellow fever with a report of no, or extremely few, cases of yellow fever among them."

Carter admitted that there was a possibility that light attacks might have occurred and passed unnoticed, unless they had given rise to yellow fever in others.

He then applied a second test. Is yellow fever ever communicated to others from cases of sickness of men who had previously had yellow fever? Men "protected by a previous attack of yellow fever" have moved about from places virulently infected into susceptible communities in the United States, hundreds of times during epidemics, and if not immune some of those men should have contracted yellow fever and developed it in an infectable but not infected place. Even if not diagnosed it should have infected mosquitoes and spread to others in whom the diagnosis would be easy. No instance of this sort was known to him; yet the evidence to the contrary had not been scrutinized carefully.

"Since we did not believe that secondary cases of yellow fever occurred—or occurred very rarely—if an outbreak occurred we would be little apt to impute conveyance of yellow fever to any sickness of indeterminate nature occurring among people who were 'protected by a previous attack of yellow fever.' "

"To use this test, then, we must depend upon the scrutiny of exposure of susceptible communities to cases of sickness of such 'protected' men who had themselves been exposed to yellow fever, and under such conditions *that other sources of exposure to the community are excluded.* Opportunity for this would rarely occur during an epidemic."

Carter goes on to cite epidemiological data as evidence against the occurrence of second cases infective to *Aëdes calopus (Stegomyia).*

"Thus, between the years 1888 and 1898, there entered Florida ports over thirty thousand people certified as 'Protected from yellow fever by previous attack or ten years' residence in an infected focus.' They came during the summer, May 1st to October 31st, from Havana, where yellow fever prevailed during this time, to Key West and Tampa—towns full of *Aëdes calopus (Stegomyia)* and of people susceptible to yellow fever. The time of passage was about eight hours to Key West, and twenty-four to Tampa. As no yellow fever developed in Florida during this period, there should have been no considerable number of secondary attacks infective to *Aëdes calopus (Stegomyia)* among these people.

"That yellow fever could be readily contracted from Havana by people susceptible to it is shown by the fact that during this time four hundred and fifty people from Havana, not certified as immune to yellow fever, yielded thirteen cases of yellow fever at a quarantine station."

2. **Rocky Mountain Spotted Fever.**—From a careful study of clinical symptoms and lesions, Wilson and Chowning (1902) considered that Rocky Mountain spotted fever was probably infectious. The sharply delimited area of prevalence, seasonal occurrence (March to July) corresponding to the tick season, lack of evidence of spread by direct contact or by food or water, absence of sex or age selection, and presence of small wounds in the skin apparently

caused by tick bites, led them to conclude that the disease was tick-borne. Their experimental work failed because they used the rabbit which is insusceptible.

3. **Poliomyelitis.**—Frost (1913) reported on his investigations of epidemics of anterior poliomyelitis in Iowa in 1910; in Cincinnati, Ohio, in 1911 and, with James P. Leake, in Buffalo and Batavia, New York, in 1912. These studies are characterized by meticulous recording of epidemiological and clinical data, with especial reference to abortive and suspected cases. In Mason City, Iowa, Frost obtained evidence of possible transmission by direct contact in an unusually high proportion of cases. He made an analysis of the apparent contagiousness of the disease, making comparisons with observations of others, notably of Hill (1910) in poliomyelitis, and of Chapin (1909) in diphtheria and scarlet fever. In the description of the Buffalo epidemic, Frost noted and commented on the fact that in rural areas the ages of those attacked tended to be higher than in metropolitan communities. He pointed out that this variation was in conformity with the theory that the quite general immunity of older persons to the disease might be specific, that is, acquired from previous unrecognized infection with the virus of poliomyelitis.

The New York epidemic of 1916 was investigated by Lavinder, Freeman, and Frost (1918) and provided much more substantial data than had been available in previous studies. To quote Maxcy (1941): "These two bulletins form a cornerstone of what is known about the epidemiology of poliomyelitis in the United States."

4. **Influenza.**—In December, 1918, after the second wave of the pandemic but before the third, Frost, Sydenstricker and their associates (1919) and Frost (1920) of the Public Health Service carried out sampling surveys of the general population in ten cities throughout the country, and in smaller cities and rural areas in Maryland. The data collected included for each *individual,* name, sex, color, age, and whether or not ill since September 1, 1918, with influenza, pneumonia, or indefinite illness; for each *case,* date of onset, duration and nature of illness, and date of death if death resulted; and for each *household,* the number of rooms occupied and the inspector's impression of economic status. The records of morbidity and mortality thus obtained, together with the official mortality statistics for influenza and pneumonia, made pos-

sible valid estimates of the real impact which the epidemic made on various age, sex, racial, and economic groups in different sections of the country.

Class 3: Epidemiological Methods Applied to Noninfectious Diseases

1. **Descriptive Study of Poisoning by Illuminating Gas.**—About 1885 in Massachusetts a movement by commercial companies to replace ordinary coal gas by a new and somewhat cheaper illuminating gas heavier in carbon monoxide called "water-gas" caused a considerable controversy. A careful report on the public health aspects of the matter was prepared in 1885 by Dr. S. W. Abbott, then secretary of the State Board of Health. The modern process prevailed but a State Gas Commission was appointed which was directed in 1888 to investigate and report all deaths (or injuries to health) from gas poisoning. The question of the relative poisonous properties of coal gas and water gas was referred for study to Mr. W. R. Nichols and Dr. W. T. Sedgwick, who found, as was expected, that water gas was much more dangerous. The mortality statistics which became available were unique for the time and were studied by Sedgwick and Schneider (1911). Prior to 1885 there had been only four deaths reported during 20 years. From 1886 to 1909 there were 1,231 deaths. A comparison with death rates from measles and scarlet fever was made showing that gas deaths promised soon to exceed those from either of these infections. It was urged by some that it was difficult to determine whether a gas poisoning death was accidental or suicidal and that gas was merely a substitution for some other means of suicide. This point was examined carefully and rejected. Among the pertinent facts was the difference in seasonal distribution between suicidal gas deaths and those classed as accidental. The seasonal distribution of the former resembled that of suicides from all causes; whereas accidental gas deaths were highest in December, when the days were shortest and lowest in July. The article concludes with a discussion of the possible dangers to health from small leaks of gas and a demand for a return to the 10 per cent limit of concentration of carbon monoxide until such time as evidence was forthcoming that a higher percentage could be used safely.

2. **Experimental Studies of Endemic Goiter.**—A series of brilliant experimental studies on endemic goiter in animals by Marine

and his associates led to success in prophylaxis of goiter in man by administration of iodine. The peculiar geographic distribution of endemic goiter had long been known and iodine therapy had been extensively used for more than a century. These workers demonstrated that iodine is a normal constitutent of the thyroid gland, that the amount varies in different animals, that variations are greatest in goitrous districts and lowest in nongoitrous, that hypertrophic and hyperplastic changes in the thyroid begin when the store of iodine falls below 0.1 per cent, and that administration of small quantities of iodine arrests this process and brings about involution of the gland. Reference is made particularly to the work on brook trout by Marine and Lenhart (1911) and Marine (1914). This is an example of an experimental study stimulated by the behavior of a disease in nature, in which groups of trout, differing as far as could be determined only as regards their food supply, were subjected to prolonged observation and pathologic study. Addition of iodine to the food prevented the disease, greatly improved the condition of goitrous fish, and pointed clearly to a method of prevention and cure of goiter in man.

4. Field Studies of Pellagra.—The exploratory study of Goldberger, Wheeler, and Sydenstricker (1918) in 1916 on pellagra in textile mill villages of South Carolina is noteworthy in at least four respects: it was the earliest extensive field study of a noninfectious disease; it was adequately controlled; it was the first systematic attempt to discover all clinically recognized cases, and it yielded significant returns. To discover cases, a house-to-house canvass was made every two weeks for several months. A dietary basis was suspected and detailed records of food consumed were obtained for each household for a fifteen-day period. An increasing supply of milk or of fresh meat was found associated, one independent of the other, with a decreasing pellagra incidence.

VIII. THEORY OF EPIDEMICS

It is not surprising that there are to be found in the American literature of the period few statistical excursions into epidemiological theory. Public health was a new profession. Populations were increasing rapidly and constantly outgrowing sanitary facilities, and the small band of epidemiologists found themselves faced with a succession of epidemics, the investigation of which could not be put off until tomorrow. Furthermore, the more dramatic discoveries of microbiology doubtless attracted to the laboratory a number of investigative minds which at a later date might have been devoted to statistical matters. In England, Brownlee commenced his studies of the epidemic curve about 1906, incidentally bringing to light a brilliant but forgotten contribution of William Farr. Hamer in the same year studied the periodicity of measles. In Germany, Mueller in 1914, and in England, Ronald Ross in 1915-1916, endeavored to describe epidemiological factors in mathematical terms. In the United States, Lotka (1912), stimulated by the publications of Ross, offered a solution for a certain system of differential equations obtained by Ross. Lotka considered also that quantitative methods could be applied with advantage to a disease not epidemic in occurrence as, for example, tuberculosis, although adequate data were not at hand. He says: "Brief reflection shows that we can apply to this case a mathematical treatment precisely analogous to that of the growth of a population; for we may think of the diseased portion of the population as a separate aggregate, into which new individuals are recruited by fresh infections, just as new individuals enter an ordinary population by procreation. On the other hand, members are continually eliminated from the aggregate, first by deaths, secondly by recoveries. On the basis of these considerations formulae can without difficulty be established between the factors enumerated above. Such general formulae, however, involve certain functions which are unknown, and the determination of which by statistical methods would at best present great difficulties."

Henry R. Carter did a great deal of serious thinking on the quantitative aspects of the balance between man and microorganisms but did not venture into extensive mathematical description. He was concerned, particularly, with an observed phenomenon, namely, the occasional spontaneous disappearance of yellow fever from regions where it was endemic and where *Stegomyia* (*Aëdes*) was abundant and active at all seasons. The following quotations are taken from his classic paper (Carter, 1919-1920) on this subject:

"Note that in such places it is not necessary to exterminate Stegomyia to eliminate yellow fever. If the number of mosquitoes be brought below the 'critical number' for yellow fever—at that place the disease will die out. Note too—that this critical number for any place will vary directly as the proportion of men immune to yellow fever to the total population.

"Thus: if with 100 cases of yellow fever introduced into a community in which all were susceptible to yellow fever, the number of Stegomyia were such that exactly 100 men would be infected from them, the disease would neither die out nor increase. This would be the critical number of Stegomyia for that place and time. With fewer mosquitoes than this, less than 100 men would be infected and the fever would die out. If more, it would increase. Now if one-quarter of the inhabitants are immune to yellow fever, obviously the same number of mosquitoes which infected 100 men before would now infect only 75—one-quarter of their bites going to immunes, and hence wasted—and the disease would die out. The number of mosquitoes required to infect 100 more men, and hence perpetuate the fever, would have to be increased by one-third above the first number.

"Obviously then this critical number, below which the Stegomyia must be brought to eliminate fever is less in a town as the proportion of susceptible people increases and more intensive work is required to eliminate it from such a community, other things being equal, than from one in which a large proportion of the population is immune."

"From the known facts of the conveyance of yellow fever, it is obvious that the conditions for the continued existence of yellow fever in a community are three: the parasites, active *Aëdes (Stegomyia) calopus,* and susceptible men; all present at the same time— the insects having access to both classes of men.

"Parasites exist only in an infected mosquito or in an infected man. They live in the mosquito only during its life, and only a short time—infective to mosquitoes—in man.

"Here, then, are two postulates:

"1. Since the parasites in the mosquito live only during the life of the host—say, ten days—no interval greater than 10 days may elapse between the date when some sick man is bitten by them, and the date when one of the mosquitoes infected by him feeds on a man susceptible to yellow fever, without the death of the parasites, and hence the extinction of yellow fever in that community.

"2. Susceptible people, then, are necessary for the continuance of yellow fever in a community. Such people must not only be present, but must be present under certain conditions of time and place with relation to the Stegomyia infected from other people with yellow fever. If in a community there be no susceptible people fulfilling these conditions, yellow fever will disappear.

"Now let us consider a community in the tropics in which yellow fever is present, Stegomyia abundant and active at all seasons, and with susceptible people. Parasites, of course, are present in those sick of yellow fever, and, since Stegomyia are active all the year round, this place will be an *endemic focus* of yellow fever.

"Obviously, if one attack of yellow fever produces in general a permanent immunity, such a community will have in time no people susceptible to yellow fever left, unless there is an introduction of such people. Yellow fever would then disappear, and, as soon as the infected mosquitoes died off (within our 10 days), the parasites would disappear and the community be free from infection. Indeed, yellow fever would doubtless disappear before there were 'no people susceptible to yellow fever left,' because, under the doctrine of chances, there would be no susceptible people left fulfilling the conditions of time and place mentioned above before there were absolutely none at all—possibly long before. Once free, it would remain free forever, unless the same three factors for conveyance are again brought together. In the natural course of events a new generation would grow up susceptible to yellow fever, susceptible immigrants move in, and Stegomyia bred to the limit; but unless the *parasite* be again introduced the community would remain free from yellow fever. In such a community—growing naturally—an epidemic would result if parasites are introduced some years after it has been free of infection, the maximum age of the natives then developing the yellow fever depending on the length of the interval of freedom.

"An immigration of susceptible people, then, is necessary for the continuation of yellow fever in a community, and if this immigration fails, or fails to fulfil certain conditions, yellow fever disappears. This mechanism I have called the 'elimination of yellow fever by failure of the human host.' "

IX. DISCUSSION AND SUMMARY

A review is presented of American Epidemiology during the period 1876-1920 with brief discussion of important concurrent events in medicine and public health which contributed to its growth.   In accordance with the concept of the period the review is restricted chiefly to the infectious diseases, and in particular to the development of knowledge and theory relating to their occurrence and spread.

The greatest advances were attributable to the application of experimental methods.   The production of disease in animals and, in notable instances, in human volunteers, under conditions which permitted measurement of a single variable, brought to epidemiology precise and exact knowledge otherwise unobtainable.   Nevertheless, to make a vertical division between experimental and field studies of the period would be to separate essential parts of the same picture.   In retrospect, at least, there was logical sequence of approach.   In Rocky Mountain spotted fever, for example, there were early clinical descriptions, followed by a comprehensive field study leading directly to experimental work which, although not immediately successful, was brilliantly so a few years later.   In yellow fever likewise a host of earlier observations, notably those of Carter and of Finlay, led to the crucial experiments of the Army Yellow Fever Commission.   As a general rule, American epidemiologists were quick to turn to the laboratory and experimental workers were stimulated and guided by field observations.

The pinnacles of the period were the establishment of two great principles, second only in importance to proof of specificity itself. These were transmission by arthropods, often from animal sources, and by healthy carriers.   American scientists made fundamental contributions to knowledge of arthropod transmission, and of existence and importance of animal reservoirs in certain diseases. Observations by Americans regarding frequency and importance of healthy carriers were also significant, but major credit for demonstration of the role of carriers goes to Europeans.

The theory of immunity from specific subclinical infection, which goes far to explain the mass phenomena of infectious diseases, also had its origin during the period.   It was probably studies on tuberculosis which first awakened the medical world to the distinction between infection and disease.   As regards acquirement of immunity without clinical attack, there were old observations on the beneficial effect of "acclimatization" on the incidence of typhoid and certain other diseases.   The relative immunity from pneumonia of native laborers after three months residence on the Isthmus of Panama is likewise a case in point.   An increasing body of data on the frequency with which healthy persons with no history of attack harbored pathogenic microorganisms led to the obvious corollary that immunity to certain diseases likewise must be widespread. The theory that this immunity is specific in origin received substantial support from studies of diphtheria. In this connection the basic work was European, but the extensive application of the Schick test, especially in New York City, demonstrated for the first time the wide distribution of antitoxic immunity and its positive association with increasing age and aggregation of population.

Certain investigations are cited to illustrate the evolution of epidemiology during the period. These relate to (1) extension of knowledge of infectious diseases of known etiology, (2) exploratory studies of diseases considered to be infectious but of unknown etiology, and (3) application of epidemiological methods to noninfectious conditions.

In the first class there are included several investigations of epidemic and endemic typhoid fever. The cause and potential modes of transmission were known, but in each local outbreak the actual vehicle had to be determined with expedition and certainty. This was not always a simple task, especially in those instances where suspicion fell upon drinking water from a supply common to all the inhabitants. In all instances it was necessary to build up circumstantial evidence incriminating a particular vehicle and to eliminate all others which might have been operative. The meticulous and convincing manner in which this was done in a very large number of epidemics is greatly to the credit of the epidemiologists of the period. Endemic typhoid presented even greater difficulties as it was necessary not only to identify the vehicles but to make an appraisal of the relative importance of each where more than one were operating in a community. Hundreds of articles were published dealing with the potentialities of the typhoid bacillus to survive outside the body. The comment may be made that only a few leaders appear to have appreciated the fact that actual sources must be determined by field studies.

In natural infections the dosage received by individuals must vary greatly and in most instances it is probably a matter of chance. The nearest approach to equivalency in dosage in diseases transmitted directly from person to person is found in the households of patients. Here also is found the nearest approximation in nature to the limits of incidence of clinically recognizable disease. The peculiar importance of this group was first taken advantage of in studies of diphtheria and scarlet fever in Providence, R. I., which dealt with such questions as immunity conferred by attack, value of hospitalization of patients, and others. The findings and methodology of these studies represent a major contribution to American epidemiology.

Early field studies of yellow fever, Rocky Mountain spotted fever, anterior poliomyelitis, and influenza are cited as examples of exploratory investigations of diseases of unknown etiology but presumed to be infectious. Descriptions of the natural behavior of these diseases gave general direction to the laboratory experiments of subsequent years—experiments which in the case of yellow fever and Rocky Mountain spotted fever led ultimately to almost complete explanation of their epidemiology, and in poliomyelitis and influenza, to significant progress toward this end.

Comment is made in the Introduction to the effect that the broadening of the term "Epidemiology," which has taken place in more recent times, making it even more inclusive than "Historical and Geographical Pathology" or "Social Pathology," has certain advantages. It may be added that modern medicine, vital statistics, and public health administration, which contributed to the growth of epidemiology in the more limited sense, at the same time furnished a larger sphere for the application of its methodology. Examples taken from the last decade of the period illustrate the profitable application of epidemiological methods to illuminating gas poisoning, endemic goiter, and pellagra, and may be taken as marking the expansion of the field of epidemiology in the United States.

Epidemiologists of the Bacteriological Era, American and other, provided for an extension of the field in two ways which are less tangible. In the first place, epidemiological description of disease was given its place as an essential part of medical knowledge. The search for differentiating features in the mass phenomena of cancer, diabetes, and other conditions has its prototype in the earlier search for definitive characteristics of influenza, measles, poliomyelitis, typhoid and other infections. A second point is the oft repeated demonstration that although in epidemiological terms the occurrence of an infectious disease is determined by dosage of a pathogen sufficient to overwhelm resistance of the human host, there are social and economic factors which may cause, augment or prevent exposure and which may raise or lower resistance. Modern studies of the relationship of these factors to the occurrence and frequency of noninfectious conditions thus received guidance and impetus from the epidemiology of the Bacteriological Era.

References

Abel, R.: 1894. Ueber die Schutzkraft des Blutserums von Diphtheriereconvalescenten und gesunden Individuen gegen tödtliche Dosen von Diphtheriebacillenculturen und Diphtheriebacillengift bei Meerschweinchen, Deutsche. med. Wchnschr. **20**: 899-902 and 936-937.

Adami, J. G.: 1899. On Latent Infection and Subinfection, and on the Etiology of Hemochromatosis and Pernicious Anemia, J. A. M. A. **33**: 1509-1514 and 1572-1576.

Albrecht, H., and Ghon, A.: 1901. Ueber die Aetiologie und pathologische Anatomie der Meningitis cerebrospinalis epidemica, Wien. klin. Wchnschr. **41**: 985-996.

Anderson, J. F.: 1912. Some Recent Contributions by the United States Public Health and Marine Hospital Service, J. A. M. A. **58**: 1748-1751.

Anderson, J. F., and Goldberger, J.: 1911. Experimental Measles in Monkeys, a Preliminary Report, Pub. Health Rep. **26**: 847-848.

—, and —: 1912. Relation of So-called Brill's Disease to Typhus Fever, Pub. Health Rep. **27**: 149-160.

Ashburn, P. M., and Craig, C. F.: 1907. Experimental Investigations Regarding the Etiology of Dengue Fever, J. Infect. Dis. **4**: 440-475.

Avery, O. T., Chickering, H. T., Cole, R., and Dochez, A. R.: 1917. Acute Lobar Pneumonia, Prevention and Serum Treatment, Monograph 7, Rockefeller Institute for Medical Research.

Brill, N. E.: 1898. A Study of Seventeen Cases of a Disease Clinically Resembling Typhoid Fever, But Without the Widal Reaction; Together With a Short Review of the Present Status of the Sero-Diagnosis of Typhoid Fever, New York M. J. **67**: 48-54 and 77-82.

Brouardel, P., and Thoinot, L.: 1905. Fiévre Typhoïde, Paris, Baillière, pp. 30-31.

Buerger, L.: 1905. Studies of the Pneumococcus and Allied Organisms With Reference to Their Occurrence in the Human Mouth, J. Exper. Med. **7**: 497-546.

Carlisle, R. J.: 1906. Two Cases of Relapsing Fever, J. Infect. Dis. **3**: 233-265.

Carter, H. R.: 1899-1900. A Note on the Interval Between Infecting and Secondary Cases of Yellow Fever From the Records of the Yellow Fever at Orwood and Taylor, Miss., in 1898, New Orleans M. & S. J. **52**: 617-636.

—: 1916-1917. Immunity to Yellow Fever, Ann. Trop. Med. **10**: 153-167.

—: 1919-1920. The Mechanism of the Spontaneous Elimination of Yellow Fever From Endemic Centers, New Orleans M. & S. J. **72**: 347-360.

Chagas, Carlos: 1909. Ueber eine neue Trypanosomiasis des Menschen, Mem. Inst. Oswaldo Cruz **1**: 159-218.

Chapin, C. V.: 1909. 27th Annual Report of the Superintendent of Health of the City of Providence, R. I., pp. 74-86.

Collins, S. D.: 1946. The Sickness Surveys: Types, History, and Some Results, in Nelson Loose-Leaf Medicine, Preventive Medicine, New York, Thomas Nelson and Sons, vol. 7, chapter 12, pp. 185-213.

Collins, S. D., Frost, W. H., Gover, Mary, and Sydenstricker, E.: 1930. Mortality From Influenza and Pneumonia in 50 Large Cities of the United States, 1910-1929, Pub. Health Rep. **45**: 2277-2328.

Conn, H. W.: 1895. The Outbreak of Typhoid Fever at Wesleyan University, 17th Annual Report of the State Board of Health of the State of Connecticut, New Haven, pp. 243-265.

Drigalski, W., and Conradi, H.: 1902. Uber ein Verfahren zum Nachweis der Typhusbacillen, Ztschr. f. Hyg. u. Infektionskr. 39: 283-300.

Evans, Alice C.: 1918. Further Studies on *Bacterium abortus* and Related Bacteria, J. Infect. Dis. 22: 576-593.

Ferry, N. S.: 1911. The Etiology of Canine Distemper, J. Infect. Dis. 8: 399-420.

Flexner, S.: 1900: Etiology of Tropical Dysentery, Philadelphia M. J. 6: 414-424.

Flexner, S., Clark, P. F., and Fraser, F. R.: 1913. Epidemic Poliomyelitis. Fourteenth note: Passive Human Carriage of the Virus of Poliomyelitis, J. A. M. A. 60: 201-202.

Flexner, S., and Lewis, P. A.: 1909. The Transmission of Acute Poliomyelitis to Monkeys. First Note, J. A. M. A. 53: 1639; Second Note, J. A. M. A. 53: 1913; The Nature of the Virus of Epidemic Poliomyelitis, Third Note, J. A. M. A. 53: 2095.

Flint, A.: 1845. Account of an Epidemic Fever Which Occurred at North Boston, Erie County, New York, During the Months of October and November, 1843, Am. J. M. Sc., n.s. 10: 21-35.

Francis, E.: 1919. Deerfly Fever or Pahvant Valley Plague. A Disease of Man of Hitherto Unknown Etiology, Pub. Health Rep. 34: 2061-2062.

Frost, W. H.: 1913. Epidemiologic Studies of Acute Anterior Poliomyelitis, Hygienic Laboratory Bulletin 90, United States Public Health Service.

—: 1920. Statistics of Influenza Morbidity, With Special Reference to Certain Factors in Case Incidence and Case Fatality, Pub. Health Rep. 35: 584-597.

—: 1927. Epidemiology, in Nelson Loose-Leaf System, Public Health-Preventive Medicine, New York, Thomas Nelson and Sons, vol. 2, chapter 7, p. 167.

—: 1938. The Familial Aggregation of Infectious Diseases, Am. J. Pub. Health 28: 7-13.

Frost, W. H., and Sydenstricker, E.: 1919. Influenza in Maryland; Preliminary Statistics of Certain Localities, Pub. Health Rep. 34: 491-504.

Glover, J. A.: 1920. Observations on the Meningococcus Carrier Rate and Their Applications to the Prevention of Cerebro-Spinal Fever, Medical Research Council, Special Report Series, No. 50, Privy Council, London, His Majesty's Stationery Office, pp. 133-165.

Goldberger, J., Wheeler, G. A., and Sydenstricker, E.: 1918. A Study of the Diet of Nonpellagrous and of Pellagrous Households in Textile-Mill Communities in South Carolina in 1916, J. A. M. A. 71: 944-949. Also Pub. Health Rep. 33: 2038-2051, 1918; 35: 648-713, 1650-1664, 1701-1714, 1920.

Harrison, R. G.: 1906-1907. Observations on the Living Developing Nerve Fiber, Proc. Soc. Exper. Biol. & Med. 4: 140-143.

Hektoen, Ludvig: 1905. Experimental Measles, J. Infect. Dis. 2: 238-255.

Hill, H. W.: 1910. Epidemiologic Study of Anterior Poliomyelitis in Minnesota, Tr. Sect. Prevent. Med. & Pub. Health, A. M. A., pp. 305-334.

—: 1911a. The Epidemiological Data, in The Mankato Typhoid Fever Epidemic of 1908, J. Infect. Dis. 9: 429-474.

—: 1911b. Report of Division of Epidemiology, 3rd Biennial Report of the State Board of Health of Minnesota 1909-1910, Minneapolis, pp. 207-208.

Howard, W. T., and Perkins, R. G.: 1901. Streptococcus Mucosus (Nov. Spec.?) Pathogenic for Man and Animals, J. M. Research, n.s. 1: 163-174.

King, W. W.: 1906. Experimental Transmission of Rocky Mountain Spotted Fever by Means of the Tick, Pub. Health Rep. 21: 863-864.

Koch, Robert: 1893. Die Cholera in Deutschland während des Winters 1892-93, Ztschr. f. Hyg. u. Infektionskr. 15: 89-165.

Koplik, H.: 1896. The Diagnosis of the Invasion of Measles From a Study of the Exanthema As It Appears on the Buccal Mucous Membrane, Arch. Pediat. 13: 918-922.

Landsteiner, K., and Popper, E.: 1909. Übertragung der Poliomyelitis acuta auf Affen, Ztschr. f. Immunitätsforsch. u. Exper. Therap. 2: 377-390.

Lanza, A. J., Higgins, Edwin, Laney, F. B., and Rice, G. S.: 1917. Siliceous Dust in Relation to the Pulmonary Diseases Among Miners in the Joplin District, Missouri, Bureau of Mines Bulletin 132, Department of the Interior, Washington, D. C., Government Printing Office.

Lavinder, C. H., Freeman, A. W., and Frost, W. H.: 1918. Epidemiologic Studies of Poliomyelitis in New York City and the Northeastern United States During the Year 1916, Public Health Bulletin 91, United States Public Health Service, pp. 1-310.

Levy, E. C., and Freeman, A. W.: 1908. Certain Conclusions Concerning Typhoid Fever in the South, As Deduced From a Study of Typhoid Fever in Richmond, Va., The Old Dominion J. Med. & Surg. 7: 315-338 and 411-426.

Loeffler, F.: 1884. Untersuchungen über die Bedeutung der Mikroorganismen für die Entstehung der Diphtherie beim Menschen, bei der Taube und beim Kalbe, Mitth. a. d. k. Gsndhtsamte, 2: 421-499.

Lotka, A. J.: 1912. Quantitative Status in Epidemiology, Nature 88: 497-498.

Love, A. G., and Davenport, C. B.: 1920. Defects Found in Drafted Men, Washington, D. C., Government Printing Office.

Lovett, R. W., and Richardson, M. W.: 1911. Infantile Paralysis, With Especial Reference to Its Occurrence in Massachusetts, 1907-10, Am. J. Dis. Child. 2: 369-406.

Manson, P.: 1878. The Development of *Filaria sanguinis hominis,* M. Times & Gaz. 2: 731.

Marine, David.: 1914. Further Observations and Experiments On Goitre (So-Called Thyroid Carcinoma) in Brook Trout (*Salvelinus fontinalis*), J. Exper. Med. 19: 70-88.

Marine, David, and Lenhart, C. H.: 1911. Further Observations and Experiments on the So-Called Thyroid Carcinoma of the Brook Trout (*Salvelinus fontinalis*) and Its Relation to Endemic Goitre, J. Exper. Med. 13: 455-475.

Maxcy, K. F.: 1941. Papers of Wade Hampton Frost, edited by K. F. Maxcy, New York, The Commonwealth Fund, p. 25.

McCoy, G. W.: 1908. Reports to the Surgeon General, Public Health and Marine Hospital Service. Plague in Ground Squirrels, Pub. Health Rep. 23: 1289-1294. (Report by Passed Assistant Surgeon G. W. McCoy, dated August 27, 1908, transmitted by Passed Assistant Surgeon Rupert Blue to Surgeon General.)

McCoy, G. W., and Chapin, C. W.: 1912. Further Observations on a Plague-Like Disease of Rodents With a Preliminary Note on the Causative Agent, *Bacterium tularense,* J. Infect. Dis. 10: 61-72.

Noguchi, H.: 1912. The Pure Cultivation of *Spirocheta duttoni, Spirocheta kochi, Spirocheta obermeieri* and *Sphirocheta novyi,* J. Exper. Med. 16: 199-215.

Norris, C., Pappenheimer, A. M., and Flournoy, T.: 1906. Study of a Spirochete Obtained from a Case of Relapsing Fever in Man, With Notes on Morphology, Animal Reactions and Attempts at Cultivation, J. Infect. Dis. **3**: 266-290.

Novy, F. G., and Knapp, R. E.: 1906. Studies of *Spirillum obermeieri* and Related Organisms, J. Infect. Dis. **3**: 291-393.

Park, W. H., and Beebe, A. L.: 1894. Diphtheria and Pseudo-Diphtheria, M. Rec. New York **46**: 385-401.

Park, W. H., and Zingher, A.: 1914-1915. Practical Applications Obtained From the Schick Reaction, Proc. New York Path. Soc., n.s. **14**: 151-158.

Reed, W., and Carroll, J.: 1902. The Etiology of Yellow Fever—a Supplemental Note, Am. Med. **3**: 301-305.

Reed, W., Carroll, J., Agramonte, A., and Lazear, J. W.: 1900. Etiology of Yellow Fever—a Preliminary Note, Philadelphia M. J. **6**: 790-796.

Reed, W., Vaughan, V. C., and Shakespeare, E. O.: 1904. Report on the Origin and Spread of Typhoid Fever in U.S. Military Camps During the Spanish War of 1898, Washington, D. C., Government Printing Office, p. 674.

Report: 1918. Trench Fever, Report of Commission, Medical Research Committee, American Red Cross. Members of the Commission: Baetjer, W., Macneal, W. J. (British), Opie, E. L., Pappenheimer, A. M., Peacock, A. D., Rapport, D., Strong, R. P., and Swift, H. L. Oxford University Press.

Ricketts, H. T.: 1906a. Studies of Rocky Mountain Spotted Fever by Means of Animal Inoculations, J. A. M. A. **47**: 33-36.

—: 1906b. The Transmission of Rocky Mountain Spotted Fever by the Bite of the Wood-Tick (*Dermacentor occidentalis*), J. A. M. A. **47**: 358.

—: 1907a. The Role of the Wood-Tick (*Dermacentor occidentalis*) in Rocky Mountain Spotted Fever, and the Susceptibility of Local Animals to This Disease—a Preliminary Report, J. A. M. A. **49**: 24-27.

—: 1907b. Further Experiments With the Wood-Tick in Relation to Rocky Mountain Spotted Fever, J. A. M. A. **49**: 1278-1281.

—: 1909. A Microorganism Which Apparently has a Specific Relationship to Rocky Mountain Spotted Fever, J. A. M. A. **52**: 379-380.

Rosenau, M. J., Lumsden, L. L., and Kastle, J. H.: 1907. Report on the Origin and Prevalence of Typhoid Fever in the District of Columbia, Hygienic Laboratory Bulletin 35, Public Health and Marine-Hospital Service of the United States.

—, —, and —: 1909. Report No. 3 on the Origin and Prevalence of Typhoid Fever in the District of Columbia (1908), Hygienic Laboratory Bulletin 52, Public Health and Marine-Hospital Service of the United States. Also Bulletins 44 and 78.

Rous, F. P.: 1910. A Transmissible Avian Neoplasm (Sarcoma of the Common Fowl), J. Exper. Med. **12**: 696-705.

—: 1911. A Sarcoma of the Fowl Transmissible by an Agent Separable From the Tumor Cells, J. Exper. Med. **13**: 397-411.

Schereschewsky, J. W., and Tuck, D. H.: 1915. Studies in Vocational Diseases, 1. The Health of Garment-Workers, 2. Hygienic Conditions of Illumination in Women's Garment Industry, Public Health Bulletin 71, United States Public Health Service.

Sedgwick, W. T.: 1893. On Recent Epidemics of Typhoid Fever in the Cities of Lowell and Lawrence Due to Infected Water Supply; With Observations on Typhoid Fever in Other Cities and Towns of Merrimack Valley, Especially Newburyport, 24th Annual Report of the State Board of Health of Massachusetts, Boston, pp. 667-704.

Sedgwick, W. T., and Schneider, Francis, Jr.: 1911. On the Relationship of Illuminating Gas to the Public Health, J. Infect. Dis. **9**: 380-409.

Smith, H. E.: 1896. A Report of the Stamford Typhoid Fever Epidemic, 18th Annual Report of the State Board of Health of the State of Connecticut, New Haven, pp. 161-179.

Smith, Theobald.: 1889. Preliminary Observations on the Microorganism of Texas Fever, M. News 55: 689-693.

—: 1896. Two Varieties of the Tubercle Bacillus From Mammals, Tr. A. Am. Physicians 11: 75-95.

Smith, Theobald and Kilborne, F. L.: 1893. Investigations Into the Nature, Causation, and Prevention of Texas or Southern Cattle Fever, Bulletin No. 1, United States Department of Agriculture, Bureau of Animal Industry, pp. 85-129.

Soper, G. A.: 1919. Typhoid Mary, Mil. Surgeon 45: 1-15.

Stecker, M. L., Frankel, L. K., and Dublin, L. I.: 1919. Some Recent Morbidity Data, 1915-17, Metropolitan Life Insurance Company.

Sternberg, G.: 1880-81. A Fatal Form of Septicaemia in a Rabbit, Produced by the Subcutaneous Injection of Human Saliva, National Board of Health Bulletin 2: 781-783.

Stiles, C. W.: 1902. New Species of Hookworm Parasitic in Man, Am. Med. 3: 777-778.

Strong and Associates: 1915. Harvard School of Tropical Medicine. Report of First Expedition to South America 1913. Members of the Expedition: Strong, R. P., Tyzzer, E. E., Sellards, A. W., Brues, C. T., and Gastiaburn, J. C. Harvard University Press.

Taylor, L. H.: 1885. The Epidemic of Typhoid Fever at Plymouth, Pennsylvania, M. News 46: 541-543 and 681-686.

Taylor, M. W.: 1858. On the Communication of the Infection of Fever by Ingesta, Edinburgh M. J. 3: 993-1004.

Warren, B. S., and Sydenstricker, E. 1916. Health Insurance, Public Health Bulletin 76, United States Public Health Service.

Welch, W. H., and Nuttall, G. H. F.: 1892. A Gas-Producing Bacillus Capable of Rapid Development in the Blood Vessels After Death, Bull. Johns Hopkins Hosp. 3: 81-91.

Wernstedt, W.: 1912. Some Epidemiological Experiences From the Great Epidemic of Infantile Paralysis Which Occurred in Sweden in 1911, Investigations on Epidemic Infantile Paralysis, Report from the State Medical Institute of Sweden to the 15th International Congress on Hygiene and Demography, Washington, 1912, State Medical Institute, Stockholm, pp. 235-267.

Wherry, W. B.: 1908. Plague Among the Ground Squirrels of California, J. Infect. Dis. 5: 485-506.

—: 1914. A New Bacterial Disease of Rodents Transmissible to Man. Pub. Health Rep. 29: 3387-3390.

Wherry, W. B., and Lamb, B. H.: 1914. Infection of Man With B. tularense, J. Infect. Dis. 15: 331-346.

Whipple, G. C.: 1908. Typhoid Fever, Its Causation, Transmission and Prevention, New York, John Wiley and Sons.

Wilson, L. B., and Chowning, W. M.: 1902. So-Called Spotted Fever of the Rocky Mountains, J. A. M. A. 39: 131-136.

Winslow, C.-E. A.: 1912. An Outbreak of Tonsillitis or Septic Sore Throat in Eastern Massachusetts, and Its Relation to an Infected Milk Supply, J. Infect. Dis. 10: 73-112.

Wolbach, S. B.: 1919. The Etiology and Pathology of Rocky Mountain Spotted Fever, J. M. Research 41: 1-197.

IV. THE TWENTIETH CENTURY—YESTERDAY, TODAY, AND TOMORROW (1920—)

JOHN E. GORDON, PH.D., M.D., F.A.P.H.A.*

THE years that centered around 1920 are appropriately taken as the beginning of the present-day era in American epidemiology. An accumulation of circumstances at that time brought an appraisal of attitudes and an assessment of method that had an important influence on the future direction of epidemiologic activities. For one thing, the rush of accomplishment that came to epidemiology with the bacteriological era had levelled off to the solid but less spectacular contributions that characterize a perfected and established scientific discipline. The opportunity to reflect and review gave assurance that what had been learned about the nature and behavior of communicable disease in the fifty years since the first discoveries of Pasteur (1822-1895) was as great as the product of all the preceding centuries. The gain was over a broad front, much more indeed than a precise knowledge of pathogenic microorganisms as the inciting factor in the infectious process.

To look back still further, five lines of approach to problems of mass disease had emerged from the new methods of thought and analysis that characterized the seventeenth century. First was the microbiologic method itself, initiated through the contributions of Kircher (1602-1680) and Francesco Redi (1620-1698); second, the study of the physical environment, based on the epidemiologic principle that filth (Emerson, 1927) is a factor in disease; third, the statistical approach (Graunt, 1676) to the analysis of cause; fourth, the methods of medical geography (Finke, 1792), to include historical and geographical pathology; and finally the study of disease in the field, as a naturally occurring phenomenon (Snow, 1855). All of these features of methodology, as applied to epidemiology, found profit in the remarkable contributions of the bacteriologic era. The sum of result was a comprehensive pattern of information about the specific causes of disease and about the nature, behavior and mode of origin of infection.

*Professor of Preventive Medicine and Epidemiology, Harvard University School of Public Health, Boston, Mass.

114

To have exploited fully the evident possibilities of microbiological methods was reasonable. That the inciting agent should have come to dominate epidemiologic activities and epidemiologic thought is also wholly understandable. But in the end, the question of why epidemics come and why they go was little better defined than before. In the minds of many, realization took form that disease was no longer being studied, but rather the parts of disease; that too frequently the parts were considered the principal phenomenon; and that in pursuit of knowledge about infectious agents, the main objective was being lost.

These ideas crystallized in the years immediately following the first World War, the years of the nineteen twenties. One influence contributing to that result was the first solid impact of a changing social order, bringing realization that cultural, economic, and social factors are important determinants of health and disease in groups of people. An unsatisfactory experience with the 1918 pandemic of influenza, and extensive outbreaks of poliomyelitis, meningococcal meningitis, and of encephalitis gave further proof that progress was not so great as many had presumed.

At any rate, in at least five centers of world medical thought, in Great Britain, Germany, France, the Scandinavian countries and America, a number of authorities at more or less the same time voiced the belief of a need to return to first principles, to study disease instead of its parts, and to search for cause broadly, in factors not limited to the agent that directly initiates the process. The unity of thought was remarkable. Americans who contributed to this view were Chapin (1928), (Flexner (1922), Frost (1928), Garrison (1923) and Hill (1922). These views gained ground, and Bayne-Jones (1931) spoke for American opinion when he said that for half a century the many sidelines of disease had been ignored, that the infectious agent was not of itself sufficient to establish a sound and convincing basis for epidemiology, and that factors other than the germ are necessary.

This movement did not originate precisely in 1920, nor in the years immediately following. Matters simply came to a head then. The return to a holistic interpretation of community disease, its consideration as a unified and total process, had been under way for a number of years. Opinion solidified, to give general appreciation that there is no single cause of mass disease, that causation involves more than the agent directly giving rise to the process, that cause lies also in the characteristics of the population attacked and in the features of the environment in which both host population and agent find themselves. The result is the modern concept of epidemiology as medical ecology and of disease as an ecologic process. This view is briefly enlarged, because it bears so strongly on the direction that current interests take.

EPIDEMIOLOGY AS MEDICAL ECOLOGY

Ecology is that biologic discipline which has to do with the mutual relationships of various living organisms in an environment, and their reaction to animate and inanimate surroundings. It is the influence of the total environment on the behavior of living things (Allee, 1949). A satisfactory balance between naturally contending species, in numbers and in activities, is seen as the principal factor that determines the maintenance and survival of one and sometimes all. This brings into play all factors affecting the well-being of the species, those of food, the physical environment, rates of reproduction, and many others. The existing state of this dynamic equilibrium determines how numerous a species is, at a particular time and place.

The stated principle, that a living thing depends for its maintenance and survival on a satisfactory balance with other existing species, holds equally for the infectious processes of man, animals, and plants. The contending species in this instance are a host and a parasite. That one is free living and one is parasitic does not alter the situation, any more than that one species is animal and one is plant, that one is large and the other small, or that one is powerful and dominant among living things, the other dependent and weak. Communicable disease is no independent relationship set apart from other life processes, nor are its problems a law unto themselves. The infectious process is a part of biology, another one of the resultant effects of an impact between a living organism and its environment. The environment itself is complex and many sided, with physical, biologic, and social components (Gordon and Augustine, 1948). As such, a disease entity is the result of no simple contest between a host and an agent of disease. A great variety of environmental factors have a part in its origin, and a balance of affairs determines the issue. Causation of disease is not a simple matter of specific agent, whether that be lead, alcohol, or the typhoid bacillus.

These considerations of disease in the individual have even more weight in the broader problems of community disease, where groups or herds of a selected host are at risk, and environment becomes still more complicated. The reasons are numerous. For instance, the frequency and behavior of one disease commonly determine what happens with another. Additionally, few localities are sufficiently isolated these days that they remain unaffected by the movements of disease in adjoining regions. Many infections with established predilection for one host species have a valency of such extent that they spread to others. Even when restricted to a single kind of host, an outbreak can have far-reaching effect on the well-being of other species, including man, through serious disturbances of established nutritional, economic, and social attributes. The epidemiologic problems of plants, of animals, and of man are considered to advantage as parts of a single discipline. An understanding of the world behavior of a disease is often necessary for satisfactory interpretation of the problems of a limited universe.

These features and others that might be developed have led many students of disease to a conviction that an ecologic interpretation offers greatest promise in defining the behavior of infection and of infectious diseases as mass phenomena affecting groups of people. Epidemiology, conceived as the scientific discipline concerned with the mass behavior of disease and injury in groups of people, thus becomes a part of human ecology; specifically, medical ecology. Health and disease, like the fundamental matters of existence and survival, are therby interpreted as the results of an ecologic interplay which is variously particular, continuous, reciprocal, or indissoluble. Disease in animals, in plants, in any living thing, is looked upon as a maladjustment of the host to the existing environment.

Because specific communicable disease is so regularly a matter of the reciprocal influence of two organisms, of a host and an infectious agent, the ecologic interpretation of these phenomena is believed best accomplished by separating the specific agents of disease from other elements of the environment. Communicable disease is thus looked upon as the result of an interaction of a triad, the members of which are a host—with man the primary concern—an agent of disease and last the intricate complex of environment. This modification of the simpler ecologic concept of an organism opposed to its environment, has the advantage that

it fits with modern medical attitudes in the classification and interpretation of disease, which is etiological in the sense of the agents
directly concerned in causation. Since etiology as a principle applies to all disease, the pattern for analysis just stated should hold
for all mass disease of human beings, whatever its origin; and for
all morbid processes, whatever the host primarily affected.

If communicable disease is a pure ecologic process, its aim is that
of all biologic processes, namely, to permit survival of both living
elements. Nature is as much concerned with the welfare of the
parasite as with that of the host. This has an important bearing
on principles designed to guide prevention and control. The practical objective is not so much to eradicate disease, as to modify it
to innocuousness.

Beyond the matter of survival, the health of an individual or of
a species represents a dominance of positive adaptations to its particular environment, either through greater numbers of positive
than negative adaptations, or because they are more heavily
weighted. Otherwise the organism can scarcely endure. Disease
from the standpoint of man is an unfavorable resultant of the
forces of ecology, the extent and seriousness of which depend upon
the kind of balance, the nature of the biologic equilibrium currently existing between human host and agent of disease. This is
in every sense a dynamic state, with the unfavorable adaptations
as they occur, to be assessed in terms of the clinical nature of the
disease that results, the number of persons affected, and the places
and duration of the process. And that endeavor is the business of
epidemiology.

The part that American workers have had in the evolution of
this concept of epidemiology as medical ecology is now to be
traced. The basic idea dates from antiquity, of a host and an
environment as fundamental factors in disease production, plus
something that the ancients called "the epidemic constitution,"
something that first became tangible through the work of Pasteur
(Dubos, 1950) and many others. A comparison of dates will show
the formal origin of bacteriology (Bulloch, 1938) and ecology
(Haeckel, 1870), at about the same time, 1875. Even then the
association of the two was delightfully and clearly presented by
Van Beneden (1876) in his little book *Animal Parasites and Messmates*. More than most men, either before or since, August Hirsch
(1817-1892) understood the intimate universe that comes from

association of insects, animals, and plants: how each influences the other, and how each is concerned in the health and disease of man.

Departing from the tradition of presenting epidemiology, disease by disease, in its clinical, historical, and geographical aspects, Müller (1914) of München defined the broad principles that determine the origins and fluctuations of infectious disease generally. The character and migration of populations were analyzed as epidemiologic factors, the physical environment received its natural emphasis, but most surprising of all he gave consideration to the social status of the host as a part of environmental influences.

As a health officer in Rhode Island, Chapin (1910) appreciated the value to disease control of the newly developing aids from the laboratory and the accumulating knowledge of infectious agents. As an epidemiologist, he sensed the increasing disproportion between field and laboratory study in elaboration of the ways by which disease is caused, for he observed (1928) that "since the development of bacteriology, many have been inclined to forget that, as it takes two to make a quarrel, so it takes two to make a disease, a microbe and its host." He gave this view practical emphasis when he said that "it is not so important to know that typhoid bacilli live in water for weeks, as it is to know that 99 per cent die in one week." With the purpose of taking stock and establishing principle, he set out to measure the relative importance of different sources of infection, of different modes of transmission. His work (Scamman, 1941) had an important influence in effecting a return to broad principles, in clarifying the carrier concept, and in general acceptance of arthropod transmission of infectious agents.

The theoretical considerations essential to an ecologic interpretation of epidemiology were formulated by Theobald Smith (1934). He was suited to the task by reason of his thorough training in biology and his broad interests in public health. He had pioneered in immunology and anaphylaxis, in sanitary water analysis, tuberculosis, and in many other fields. The Third International Microbiologic Congress, in striking a medal in his honor, called him a "student of disease." That he was when he translated epidemiology in terms of ecology. Infectious disease was presented as a manifestation of parasitism, an interplay between a host and an infectious agent. He analyzed the life cycle of parasites and described aberrant and incomplete cycles of parasitism. Having presented the direct association between host and parasite, he summarized those factors which determine survival of the parasite, and govern its movements from host to host.

Multiple Causation of Mass Disease

To recognize disease as the resultant of ecologic forces within a dynamic system made up of an agent of disease, a host and an environment, is to lend aid in clarifying the concept of cause. Causality rests in all three elements, in varying degree according to the individual circumstance, often with one or another feature dominant, but by no means the same one regularly. In relation to mass disease, cause has to do with the forces that both create and maintain a situation, and thus with the origin and the course that disease takes in population groups. The factors are commonly many and diverse (MacLeod, 1926).

The theory of multiple causation is not new to medicine nor to science. In both the general field, and in medicine, fashions in scientific thought—and they do exist—have brought a return to earlier concepts, that natural phenomena arise out of the complex situations in which they occur, and that many elements of that situation affect them. For the physical sciences, where precision and the ability to measure exceed most others, the eminent theorist Niels Bohr (1950) has analyzed this approach to causality in terms that are suggestively useful for biologic processes. For biology itself, Jennings (1930) has stated the fallacy of the single cause to be the commonest error of science; and Spence (1950) writing recently states his intent to view etiology in its literal sense, to include the personal and environmental circumstances leading to infection.

Etiology in Disease of the Individual

A knowledge of disease in its individual prototype commonly aids understanding of the mass phenomenon. Etiology may be said to express the sum of knowledge regarding causes. In former years a common division was of direct inciting causes and predisposing causes. From this primary separation an imposing collection of terms came into use, with etiology conceived as immediate, primary, secondary, remote, proximate, specific, ultimate, and others. Etiologic factors, conditions, causes, and influences were specified, and these in turn categorized as contributing, inciting, predisposing, and precipitating. The result was a jumble of ideas about causality that often lacked ready definition and sometimes meaning. A principal weakness was the assumption of a fixed pattern or mosaic, with different elements in ordered relation to each other. This attitude is in violation of biologic principle, for the natural phenomena of living things are dynamic, and consequently cause is variable. The search for a simplified concept led to emphasis on the most tangible and direct feature, which is the agent of disease. Thus etiology came to be viewed progressively as a function of the infectious agent in communicable disease, of arsenic and other chemicals in poisonings and intoxications, of cold in certain traumatic injuries, and a lack of vitamins in specified manifestations of inanition. A comparison of textbooks of this and the preceding generation shows this transition. The gain was an added preciseness about a part of causality. The loss was in diminished appreciation that many factors were concerned in causation, and that the inciting agent was not necessarily the primary cause of a disease process, in the sense of being the main or most important factor.

Causality of Mass Disease

The main concern here is with mass disease, with the cause of pathologic manifestations as they affect populations, and primarily human populations, rather than with disease as an abstract phenomenon or a problem of the individual. In some ways the material provided by this broadest example of the action of a morbid process has advantage over disease as it occurs in the cell, in a tissue or organ, or even in the individual. The core problem is not with the specific causes of a particular illness, nor of a specific outbreak, but rather with what makes it possible for disease to become established in a population and epidemics to prevail among people.

When disease is viewed in terms of its mass manifestations, something more is required of a concept of causality than the means by which the process comes into being. An infectious agent, in attacking populations, sometimes gives no more than an isolated case. Uncommonly, and at the other extreme, an epidemic occurs and yet both events may be temporary, with the disease subsiding, to disappear for long periods or in that region perhaps permanently. Under other circumstances, the infection becomes firmly established as a fixed feature of the invaded population, but again variably, sometimes at a regular endemic level, more commonly with irregular or periodic fluctuations in incidence, even to epidemic proportions. Severity of effect varies as much as numbers attacked, so that influenza sometimes occurs as a mild though extensive process with no deaths, as in the American Army outbreak of 1943 in Britain (Gordon, 1949), or as a 1918 pandemic with thousands of deaths (Jordan, 1927) (Vaughan, 1921). Cause in relation to mass disease thus includes additionally, consideration of the reasons for these fluctuations as they occur in time, in place, and in persons attacked.

The forces associated with origin, and those concerned with the course and extent that a crowd disease takes, can, of course, be conceived as independent matters, in analogy with etiology and pathogenesis in disease of the individual. However, the pattern of epidemiologic behavior and the origin of the process are so largely determined by the initial ecologic situation that they are inseparable concepts.

The concept of causality of mass disease on an ecologic basis had its origin in observations of infectious disease. This was a natural circumstance, in that the sole concern of epidemiology for many years was with that class of morbid processes. Most of the principles that govern disease as a mass phenomenon and the technics for its study are from that source. The infections are suited to the purpose of defining ecologic relationships for they present a direct example of one living organism acting with another in a common environment. The adaptations of both have been closely studied over long periods. As the epidemiologic method came to be applied to other mass diseases (Goldberger, Wheeler, and Sydenstricker, 1918), and to mass injuries (Gordon, 1949) as well, the same general scheme of a holistic interpretation of cause and course was found applicable. The basic elements of agent of disease, host, and environment are now examined, with the purpose of developing a general pattern for analysis of cause.

Agent of Disease.—Recognized disease agents as a class include substances of physical, chemical, and biological nature. Those of nonliving nature are often as clearly active in production of mass disease as are pathogenic microorganisms in the infections. Agents of disease act sometimes through their presence, or presence in excess amounts, as with lead or the typhoid bacillus; and sometimes through a deficiency, as with niacin in pellagra or a hormone in endocrine disorders. Consequently, disease is to be recognized (Galdston, 1942) either as a positive or a negative phenomenon.

As already stated, the separation of the agent of disease from other features of the environment is artificial and for convenience, as a means of fitting an ecologic system of disease origin to the accepted interpretations implanted to such advantage in modern medicine. The simpler fundamental ecologic system of two elements, an organism and its environment, provides a practical means for assaying cause in instances where specific knowledge of an agent is lacking, as in the epidemiology of cancer.

Host Factor.—The host factor in causation has increasing attention these days, both in relation to individual disease and to mass disease. Too frequently, however, it is viewed as an abstract or composite quality, with insufficient differentiation of its parts and still less attention to measurement and evaluation of the constituents that comprise the complex.

Contribution by the host to causation of disease is first through inherent characteristics which are variously anatomic and physiologic, genetic and developmental, and in respect to age, sex, race, and other. Acquired host characteristics are a second consideration. The specific immunity that develops from infection is the most evident and the best understood, but other acquired features have a broader influence, since they act not only in respect to infections, but in mass diseases generally, and in mass injuries. Metabolic and anatomic changes brought about in a host by a variety of other disease conditions, which range from psychiatric and mental disorders to fractures, commonly stand in causal relation to a second mass disease. The susceptibility to infection that follows diabetes is a classical example. Additionally, the long-term biochemical and physiological adaptation of populations called forth by the stimulus of environment is clearly active in determining the frequency of some diseases, the current aging of populations in relation to degenerative and neoplastic conditions being an illustration.

Environment.—Environment is a composite of many elements. It is more than the natural surroundings of a region; it includes all external conditions which have an effect on the life and development of an organism. The universe of living things, man

and all others, enters just as directly into what constitutes environment as do the more evident inanimate physical features by which
the several parts of the world are so commonly distinguished from
each other.   The manifold influences exerted by environment on
the origin and course of mass disease are interpreted to advantage
by separating these many features into the three broad categories
of a biologic environment, a physical environment, and a social
component.

Of the three, the physical surroundings of man have always had
full emphasis; and to a limited extent the idea persists that this is
the whole of environment.   Weather, climate, soil, and terrain are
such evident factors that an original search for cause in telluric
and meteorologic sources was logical.   When the discovery of
specific agents explained more rationally the behavior of cholera,
plague, and so many other diseases, the action once attributed
directly to the physical environment was turned to an improved
understanding of how these environmental forces affected host and
parasite, contributed to insanitary conditions, and thereby affected
the nature and persistence of disease.

The biologic component of environment can be taken to include
the universe of living things that surrounds man, all else than man
himself.   Epidemiologic influences of the biologic environment are
within two principal areas, of which the first is the activities of
plants and animals as reservoirs of infectious agents, and the second, as vectors of disease.   The relationship is broader.   Repeated
evidence is to be had of direct action by some living thing on one
or other member of the host-parasite complex involved in a specific
disease.   Sometimes the resistance of the human host is favorably
or adversely altered, and sometimes it is the activity of the agent
that is inhibited or enhanced.

The social component of environment is that part which results
from the association of man with his fellow man.   The preferred
term would be cultural environment, were it not for the varying
interpretation of the word culture in different lands and languages.
What is intended within the stated concept is something more than
social environment, in the strict sense of having to do with society
as an organic or organized unit composed of persons within the
community.   Since economic life so largely influences social existence, that is included.   The content is also of those environmental
influences which enter by reason of the attainments, beliefs, cus-

toms, traditions, and like features of a people. Thus, the epidemiologic factors within the social environment range from housing to food supply; and from education to the provisions made for medical care.

The concept of multiple causation does not discount the specificity of mass disease, whether the agent is arsenic, cold, or a pathogenic microorganism. It is what Winslow (1948) expressed when he spoke of the tubercle bacillus as not *the* cause of tuberculosis, but one of the causes. The ecologic approach to mass disease requires that the agent be integrated into the larger fabric of the environment and that the full answer to causality include as well the qualities possessed by the host; this despite full recognition of the essential role of the agent as the direct incitant.

Identification of Multiple Factors

Present-day epidemiology stresses the importance of the agent in disease causation, largely by reason of the better methods and the greater ease with which that factor is measured and appraised.

Interest in the host is along narrower lines; for the infections, primarily in specific immunity, and for much the same reason, that serologic and immunologic technics are readily available and exact. Resistance to infection is recognized as the sum total of body mechanisms which interpose barriers to the progress of invasion by infectious agents (Am. Pub. Health Assn., 1950). There are two main divisions. Immunity (ibid.) is resistance associated with antibodies or specifically developed tissue response for a specific disease. Inherent insusceptibility (ibid.) or autarcesis (Aycock, 1929), the second major component, is an ability to resist disease independently of antibodies or specifically developed tissue response; it commonly rests in anatomic or physiologic characteristics of the host; it may be genetic or acquired; permanent or temporary. For every mass disease, the make-up of a population and the inheritance and constitution of the individuals composing the group, have a part in determining origin and outcome. For the infections this consideration ranks with immunity, and yet it is much less appreciated. For other mass diseases and for injuries it is the whole of host factor.

As for environment, too much of evidence on its action in mass disease is empiric.

Scientific activity has always been conditioned more by available methods for study than by the relative importance of problems. The disproportionate emphasis on host and environment in causality of mass disease is suggestively due not so much to inadequate appreciation of their significance as to lack of quantitative method. The currently increasing concern with these matters would seem to be the result of a steady accomplishment in remedying existing deficiencies. American contributions date from Chapin.

By use of simple but carefully recorded data of the Providence, R. I., Health Department, Chapin and later Pope (1926) measured such determining factors in community disease as age, sex, and race. Chapin developed field technics whereby the family was the unit of epidemiologic study, and he introduced the secondary attack rate within families as a means of measuring the spread of infection. Wade Hampton Frost contributed more to quantitative method than any other American epidemiologist, through his studies on poliomyelitis (1913), the common cold (1932), and tuberculosis (1933); and through developing the modified life table technic and the index case concept. Aycock by contrast is more the biologist than the statistician. Many will think of him as an epidemiologist of a single disease, poliomyelitis, but his interests have ranged throughout the infections and they have centered consistently on principle. As one of the first in this country to work with viruses, he contributed to knowledge of the virus of poliomyelitis, but more to an understanding of what it does and how it acts in populations of people. He defined seasonal (Aycock, 1945), racial and geographic relationships, measured the frequency of inapparent infections and identified qualities of the host which determine the eventual result as disease or immunizing infection.

A principal feature of the modern concept of mass disease as an ecologic phenomenon is the weight accorded social factors in disease causation. The problem of causality is more than biological. Exploitation of the relationship between social and biological factors is inhibited as much as anything by the failure of the social sciences to provide data comparable to those of the biological sciences, data susceptible to statistical analysis. The increasing association of workers in the two fields in attack on problems of mass disease should have the beneficial result of developing common methods and a common means of approach.

Multiple Causation in Practice

A concept of multiple causation was a natural consequence of viewing mass disease holistically, as an ecologic phenomenon. The basic scheme just given for examination of agent, host, and environment, as each contributes to the end result, serves to demonstrate principle. For practical application in the field, this simple scheme is enlarged to advantage through appropriate subdivisions of the three cardinal elements. The test of its applicability to analysis of cause is to demonstrate that it applies to all mass diseases and to the various distributions and frequencies that they show, a matter clearly beyond the scope or the purpose of this presentation. An illustration in respect to one disease, malaria, and one kind of distribution, the epidemic, has value in bringing out principle.

As a country, Romania had long had tertian malaria of irregular distribution, with the disease absent in the Transylvania highlands, relatively mild and geographically discontinuous along the great river valleys, curiously absent in the delta of the Danube, and of prominence only along the southern Black Sea coast. When the delta was occupied in 1917-1918 by Bulgarian and Turkish troops, it became a hotbed of malaria (Zotta, 1932). Malaria increased throughout other large areas of the country to become truly epidemic. The agent of disease was the determining factor. *P. falciparum,* not previously present, was imported by foreign troops.

Greece is heavily infected with malaria, as much so as any country outside the tropics. From time to time epidemic proportions are reached, the "endemic-epidemic" malaria described by Balfour (1936). Mass exchanges of population after World War I led to the settlement in 1922 of more than a million nonimmune immigrants in some 1,400 new villages in malaria-seeded Macedonia. Malaria was greatly increased over a long period, the primary factor in this instance being an altered constitution of the host population.

Greece provides still another kind of situation. After World War II, the general destruction, the displacement of people, undue rainfall, and insufficient food and drugs produced epidemics in places such as Athens where malaria had almost disappeared (Boyd, 1949). The outbreaks in this instance were related to an altered social and physical environment.

In 1940, *A. gambiae* was reported in the port of Natal on the east coast of Brazil. This mosquito, common in Africa but previously not recognized in the Americas, is one of the more efficient vectors of malaria. Soon thereafter, Natal experienced an explosive outbreak of malaria, which spread to other areas and was followed by a series of epidemics over the next ten years, until control measures eventually eliminated *A. gambiae*. These unique epidemics were explained (Soper and Wilson, 1943) by the presence of a vector newly introduced by man in the course of intercontinental traffic; and the primary cause was an alteration of the biologic environment. The examples cited reveal two principles.

The first principle is that similar instances of disease and similar epidemics may arise from dissimilar causes. The primary factor in causation, in the sense of the most important factor, may be variously the agent of disease, the host, or some one of the three components of the environment.

Although one or the other of the elements of the ecologic triad may dominate a situation, none of the examples cited show one element alone responsible for the malaria in a population or for the course the epidemic took. Causation is a product of all three, although the contributions by each expectedly vary. The second principle therefore follows, that in the analysis of cause all factors entering into disease production and disease distributions necessarily are kept in view at the same time and each in relation to the other.

Quantitative Causality of Mass Disease

The variety of factors that enters into the fabric of cause, and the differences in degree to which the several factors act, require in any given situation that they be quantitated, whereby independent variables are isolated from the dependent and assessed in relation to the observed total effect. The progress made in modern statistical method is such that the difficulty is not in that field. The need is for better data on host and environment. The main source at present is in the biological and sanitary sciences. The facts there obtained need to be enlarged by usable information from the social sciences, social anthropology and human genetics, where definition of variables and means for measuring them are all too loose.

An approach to understanding of mass disease through multiple causality gives promise of equalizing the emphasis so long placed on the agent. It should aid in integrating the various mass diseases of man into the general medical and social interests of communities, rather than considering them as things individual and set apart.

THE EPIDEMIOLOGIC METHOD

In search for an improved prevention and a better clinical management, workers in the communicable diseases have long recognized three fundamental approaches to knowledge. Information is first to be had from bedside study of the sick individual. This is clinical investigation. Second, and as the principal reliance of modern medicine, important results originate under the controlled conditions of laboratory experiment. The third method is epidemiological, through observation of disease as it occurs under natural conditions in whole populations. It is to be understood that the epidemiologic method is in no sense offered as a substitute, either for clinical study which is clearly the point of departure in any investigation of disease or for the experimental method. This third method, however, has many times supplemented the other two; and has to its independent credit some of the outstanding discoveries in communicable and other disease.

The choice of method of study is often determined by the level at which investigation is directed. For disease of a cell or of a tissue, experimental methods are about the only practical approach. When the level of interest is an organ, investigation by experiment may still be preferred, with clinical procedures an alternative. Clinical study finds its main application at the level of the individual, but again not to the exclusion of experiment. By definition, the field methods of epidemiology come into play where the unit of study is a population; and are there the principal reliance, supplemented to an extent by the newer technics of experimental epidemiology. Because disease is a broad biological process, a rounded study commonly makes use of all three methods, clinical, experimental, and epidemiological.

More general use of the epidemiologic method has been limited as much as anything by a common interpretation of its content as restricted to simple incidence and prevalence of disease (Gordon and le Riche, 1950) and sometimes even those two features are not clearly differentiated. Together they make up an elementary epidemiology as fundamental as the determination of temperature, pulse, and respiration in clinical medicine. A second larger objective is to refine and extend the data of incidence and prevalence in derivation of cause, through comparing different divisions of a population exposed to different environmental conditions. A third feature of epidemiologic procedure is the design of experimental field studies, sometimes to test the validity of laboratory observations, but more commonly in search of further evidence to support hypotheses of cause as derived from naturally occurring disease. The analogy with clinical methods is evident. Experimental procedure is also incorporated. Epidemiology thus serves two main purposes, first as a means by which the scientific method is applied to the practice of public health and the control of disease; and second, as an instrument for research.

It is possible to distinguish four general stages in the evolution of method for study of mass disease. Although each represents a departure in attitude and approach, what really took place was a progressive refinement and enlargement of a basic scheme which was the Hippocratic doctrine of observe, record, and reflect. A brief statement of what happened from the beginning therefore aids in understanding epidemiological method as it is today.

A Descriptive Procedure

The study of disease in the field was for many centuries primarily descriptive. Added exactness came through introduction of systems for the collection of demographic data (Graunt, 1676); and through vital statistics came a means to assay more closely the observed events in the life and the health of people.

The Comparative Method

The historical-geographical concept of field study was formalized by Finke in 1792. It dominated practice until the end of the nineteenth century, reaching its finest development with Hirsch (1883-1886). Attention was almost wholly with epidemics. As such, the study of disease in nature was in large part retrospective, often instituted after the process was well under way, and many times after it had ended. The chief aim was to describe the form that biologic processes took as mass disease, rather than an attention to their dynamic relationships. The main gain was an extension of interest beyond the event itself, to bring comparison with similar events at other times and in other places. The result was progress in understanding cause of origin and course.

An Analytical Discipline

What Panum (1847) and Snow (1855) and numerous others brought to field practice midway in the nineteenth century was an active participation and a personal observation of what was taking place as it occurred. This marked a transition from study of fixed and finished events to a concern with the dynamic relationships of transmissible disease. The broad interests that characterized these early field investigations were restricted before long to a narrower concern with sources of infection and modes of spread, by reason of the powerful potentialities that arose from the rapidly developing sciences of microbiology. A practical result, however, was an improved understanding of disease processes and perfected measures for control, that so limited the frequency of epidemics as to give time for the study of individual cases and for evaluation of endemic distributions of disease. The significance of these simpler situations as the precursor of epidemics was realized. As a result, epidemiological investigations became a formal part of health department activities and an operational procedure. A principal American stimulus to this end was from Chapin. Leadership came also from the old Hygienic Laboratory of the Public Health Service through Rosenau (1899-1909) and McCoy (1915-1937), and from W. H. Park in New York City. The movement was evident in many states and cities, for instance in Minnesota, Massachusetts, and New York, where a succession of distinguished workers has maintained an epidemiologic tradition established, respectively, by Hibbert W. Hill, by Walter H. Brown and by Edward S. Godfrey, Jr.

The accumulating knowledge of epidemiological theory and the increasing use of statistical methods led progressively to a turn of epidemiology from a descriptive and comparative procedure to an analytical discipline. If one American is to be singled out as contributing most forcefully to this change, he is W. H. Frost. In his teaching, through his students, and by his own contributions, Frost developed means for quantitating mass phenomena of disease and for measuring the biologic attributes of disease as evidenced in populations of people. Once established as an analytical discipline the way was clear for epidemiology to make full use of the technical methods originating from other medical and biological sciences, and to perfect field methods of study.

The Pattern for Field Study.—Field study, as it has developed in this present era, is based on the principle of bringing clinical and laboratory procedures to the study of disease in the homes of people, as a unified and coordinated effort along with field observations. Field data are thereby enlarged, and acquire added exactness. The chief gain is that a single disease situation is studied in nature and concurrently by the three primary methods of medical investigation, with each contributing to the other.

Clinical Contribution.—Classical field method has itself changed little in the evolution of the combined approach. The family continues as the unit of study. The investigation pertains to a prescribed and defined universe. The field of action is the observation of inter-related effects of an environment and a host. What has happened is that by bringing modern clinical methods to the field, disease is studied in all degrees of severity. Latent infection receives the same careful attention so commonly reserved for more desperate illness. Clinical interpretation of a disease process is thus more nearly related to the total of its possible manifestations. Because disease is searched for, instead of discovered only as the patient seeks medical care, the beginnings of disease are better seen than in most other situations.

Laboratory Participation.—Field method has profited greatly through incorporation of laboratory technics as an integral part of the procedure. This has followed two directions. In the first instance, microbiological and other methods of precision have been used in direct evaluation of the varied attributes of host and environment, through sampling such diverse things as the air of rooms and the pus from lesions, in determining the quality of foods, and in measuring climate and weather. Another signal advance is the increasing practice of extending field observations to the experimental laboratory, through materials collected in the field. The reverse is also done, in that results of laboratory experiment are taken to the field for practical test, either to determine that they apply to man, or more particularly that they apply to man as he functions under natural conditions.

Team Effort.—This new kind of field study has led to changes in organization for field investigation. The things now done in the field are manifestly beyond the competence of a single individual. Many data are better collected by specialists in disciplines other than medicine. Plans are on a broader scale. The days of the lone investigator with an objective limited to sources of infection have passed into history; and for the reason that both are outmoded. Operational epidemiology as practiced by health departments has become a team effort. The basic elements of the team are drawn from representatives of epidemiology, the laboratory, and from clinical skills, to include those of the veterinarian and the dentist. The work of the day is largely done by the public health nurse, and by sanitarians and other technically trained assistants. The entomologist, the sanitary engineer, the geneticist, and all manner of specialists in both biological and social sciences may participate according to the problem at hand. The Communicable Disease Center of the Public Health Service, with interests that are both operational and investigative, gives illustration of an organization and staffing based on the principle of teamwork.

The Field Survey.—Despite these changes in viewpoint and method, field study continued for many years to be pretty much an emergency measure. To be sure, activities expanded from a sole concern with epidemics to include the rest of the process, as represented by endemic disease. The finer details of sporadic and single cases were studied, but not in systematic approach to community disease. The increasing emphasis on epidemiology as an analytical discipline, the diversity of skills brought into the field, the growing familiarity of field workers with the virtues of the experimental method, together with interests aroused through attention to endemic disease were factors which led to a new form of field study.

The field survey seeks to determine the frequency of a disease in a whole population at a specified time. This is cross section study and determines prevalence. The common use of the method is to assess the health of a community under usual conditions, as distinguished from study and control of an epidemic. Examples include the survey of chronic diseases in Massachusetts (Bigelow and Lombard, 1933), the Hagerstown, Maryland, studies (Sydenstricker, 1930), and the comprehensive National Health Survey (Perrott, Tibbitts, and Britten, 1939) of 1935. The method has had wide application in subsequent years, either as a general health survey or with interest in a single condition, sometimes a communicable disease (Edwards, 1940), sometimes a nutritional deficiency (Milam and Anderson, 1944), and recently diabetes in a New England town (Wilkerson and Krall, 1947).

The Field Review.—To expand this kind of field investigation into long-term study, with the purpose to determine incidence rather than prevalence, was a logical progression. The two methods may be distinguished by terming the cross-section prevalence study a field survey, and designating the long-term incidence study a field review.

Actually, the field review marked the introduction of experimental principle into field studies. Instead of observations on what had happened or was happening, field study became prospective. A design of experiment was possible; data were collected according to preformed plan, with conditions defined and constants established. Studies on syphilis (Clark and Turner, 1942) in the Eastern Health District of Baltimore and on tuberculosis in Tennessee (Puffer, et al., 1942) illustrate method and principle for chronic infection; scarlet fever in Romania (Schwentker, Janney, and Gordon, 1943) for an acute communicable disease. The main usefulness of the method became apparent as chronic noninfective diseases were included among epidemiological interests. The inherent nature of these conditions makes long-term observations essential. The Framingham heart study (Dawber, Meadors, and Moore, 1951) is designed to extend over 25 years. An ultimate understanding of rheumatoid arthritis (Lewis-Faning, 1950), cancer (Reed, 1949), and many other problems of mass pathology would seem to rest on similar procedure.

Experimental Approach

An attempt to define the general laws and principles of mass disease by experimental means was a logical step in the transition that science experienced generally, as it progressed from descriptive and comparative method to experiment. The methods of experimental pathology are to be distinguished from those of experimental epidemiology. Experimental pathology deals with disease in the experimental animal as represented by individuals or collections of individuals. The dose of the infectious agent is measured and the mode of transmission is unnatural. Experimental epidemiology, by contrast, is concerned with disease as a manifestation of whole populations of experimental animals, considered as a unit; and with an epidemic as a single broad biologic process. The mode of transmission is natural and dosage is not quantitated. The purpose of experimental pathology is to define some specific feature of the infectious process, such as the microbial agent, the route of transmission, or pathogenesis. The aim of experimental epidemiology is to determine the factors responsible for the rise and fall of epidemics, what initiates an outbreak and where and how an infectious agent remains dormant for varying periods between epidemics. Technics are developed for the production of epidemics. Model epidemics then serve in study of isolated factors in epidemic causation.

By these methods, genetic and immunological characteristics of the herd as a host have been investigated by Webster (1946), nutritional influences by Schneider (1946); and similarly various physical and social factors of the environment, each treated as independent variables with other important factors held constant.

The experimental approach to mass disease has the advantage of providing better controls than are possible in disease of man under natural conditions. A disadvantage rests in the inability to reproduce under laboratory conditions the climatic, meteorological, and other environmental conditions which so greatly influence the spread of infection, and the genesis of diseases that are not communicable. Experimental conditions cannot always be determined or controlled to assure that results reflect situations associated with natural epidemics. There is a further consideration, common to all experimental study, that the effect exhibited by animals reacting to animal pathogens is not translated with surety in explanation of the epidemiological problems of man. The results of experimental epidemiology need to be referred back to the field for test under natural conditions.

Experimental epidemiology offers promise in testing the assumptions and hypotheses that arise from field and statistical studies of natural epidemiological events. As a technical procedure much remains to be developed. Application thus far has been only to the communicable diseases primarily, leaving largely unexplored by these methods of grouped animal behavior such suggestively worthwhile fields as the poisons of industry, cancer, and mental and emotional disorder.

Trends in Methodology

The epidemiologic method as now applied to operational and research ends can reasonably expect future additions by way of the biological sciences upon which it rests. The greater potential contribution is from the social sciences. There is a growing inclination for social and biological scientists to work together. A completely satisfactory holistic interpretation of mass disease requires a better evaluation of social factors than now exists.

As noninfective diseases and injuries became a part of epidemiology, the principles established in the study of the acute infections were applied to these new problems. This was both sound and reasonable. Experience has demonstrated, however, that technical method cannot be so freely transferred. A review of methodology in chronic disease has the attention of a number of workers, with the purpose of determining patterns of study better suited to the individual requirements of these fields.

The tools of a newer biometry have been much used during the past decade in the analysis and efficient design of laboratory experiments, particularly in agriculture and pharmacology. Appreciation is developing (Ipsen, 1950) that the multifactorial experiments that nature conducts in the production of mass disease are also amenable to biometric analysis, but retrospectively and in assay of multiple causation.

The concept of an epidemiology of health introduced by Merrell and Reed (1949) suggests the usefulness of complementarity in an approach to causality, through attention to both fractions of a population, the sick and the well.

Many years ago Theobald Smith stressed comparative epidemiology, the study of naturally occurring disease among wild and domestic animals, as a fruitful means for deriving epidemiologic principle. The growing interest of veterinarians in epidemiological matters and the numbers acquiring training in its methods are reasons to anticipate a revived interest.

More than a hundred years ago the Epidemiological Society of London expressed its interest in epidemic diseases of plants as a source of information on epidemiologic principle and theory. There are many common features in communicable diseases of animals and plants as for example, transmission by arthropods.

Physicians have nevertheless continued to study their diseases and botanists theirs, with little exchange of information or pooling of interests.

THE COURSE OF EVENTS SINCE 1920

The historical record of a subject or of an era is something more than a simple narration of events. If medicine is to be put into a proper perspective, if full profit is to be had from history as a guide to the future, then the greater concern is with the forces that brought events into being rather than with the details of what happened. These are the reasons for the attention just given to epidemiological theory, and to epidemiological practice as shown in an evolving method.

In setting out now to present the tangible accomplishments of American epidemiology for the period 1920-1950, events are considered as they relate to three fields of interest. The first area has to do with additions to knowledge in the classical epidemiology of the communicable diseases. The second is the means by which epidemiological facts and epidemiological methods have been applied to social ends and an improved public health practice. The third deals with the advances of epidemiology as a profession.

Mass Pathology of the Communicable Diseases

The number of advances in the epidemiology of the infectious diseases is so great that an orderly record is scarcely possible without some systematic scheme of presentation. A primary relation to one or other member of the ecologic triad of agent, host, and environment is found convenient.

The Infectious Agent

The contributions of early American microbiologists were by no means negligible, but for many years Europe was the chief source of bacteriological advances. The effect evidenced on epidemiology in this country was in large part indirect and limited. About 1920, when America began to take its place among world leaders in microbiological research, the progress made in that field was reflected in heightened epidemiological activities, best evidenced perhaps among the virus diseases.

Virus Diseases.—Viruses had been identified long before 1920, but they still were mysterious things, thought to cause a goodly number of diseases but rarely so proved. If microbiologists may be said to have learned the virus trade by way of the variola virus, epidemiological development was through yellow fever. The investigations of the International Health Division of the Rockefeller Foundation (Strode, 1951) began in 1916. Since then, they have reached into fourteen countries and three continents. The virus of yellow fever was isolated in the course of field studies in Africa (Stokes, Bauer, and Hudson, 1927). The problem was then taken up in the laboratories of the Foundation in New York City, where a long series of studies gave understanding of the biological nature of the infectious agent. The development of a vaccine was one of the more important contributions. From time to time, results from the laboratory were returned to the field for test, and in the case of the vaccine for clinical trial. Laboratory and field investigations developed concurrently, to give definition of geographical areas involved in yellow fever, to add the concept of jungle yellow fever to that of key city distribution, and to establish practical measures for prevention and control of the disease as a world problem. For the first time in epidemiological practice, a full association of allied scientific disciplines was brought to those of medicine. The results of these studies rank high among scientific accomplishments of this modern period; they have equal value as a pattern for field study of a disease through team effort.

The disease mumps has far less clinical significance than yellow fever but biologically the attraction is equally great. In military practice (Gordon and Kilham, 1949) it is an important disease because of the frequency with which it occurs and the prolonged period of disability. At any rate, mumps has become one of the better studied virus diseases (Enders, 1945), serving as a medium for the development of principle and method in both laboratory (Henle et al., 1950) and field (Habel, 1951).

The demonstration in 1940 of at least two kinds of influenza virus (Francis, 1940) set off a series of studies that have been among the more fruitful in the virus field. The common cold (Smillie, 1940) received new attention, a wartime commission on acute respiratory diseases (Dingle et al., 1943) had interest in the whole broad field, and primary atypical pneumonia (MacLeod, 1943) was recognized as a new and relatively prevalent disease.

Infectious hepatitis was rescued from the limbo of quasi-infections to be established as a communicable disease (Havens, 1945)

(Neefe, Gellis, and Stokes, 1946) that frequently occurs in epidemic proportions (Gauld, 1946). Homologous serum jaundice or serum hepatitis was recognized for the first time (Sawyer et al., 1944) (Oliphant, Gilliam, and Larson, 1943).

Interest has continued to center on poliomyelitis (National Foundation for Infantile Paralysis, Collected Reprints, 1939-1949), one of the first diseases of man of demonstrated viral origin. The Coxsackie group of viruses (Dalldorf and Sickles, 1948) are a recent and healthy by-product.

A catalogue of activities among virus diseases is beyond the purposes of this presentation. The intent is to demonstrate the wide range of infections studied. So definite did knowledge become that the infectious agent of a disease was no longer recorded, for example, as "a filtrable virus" but as the virus of mumps. A further result was to crystallize epidemiologic interests (Harvard Symp., 1940), so that the study of virus diseases is one of the more active fields in present-day practice.

Rickettsial Diseases.—Of all major classes of infections, the rickettsial diseases come closest to being the product of American investigation. The name rickettsia stems from the American discoverer (Wilder, 1950) of this group of microorganisms. The fundamental contributions on typhus and Rocky Mountain spotted fevers belong to the preceding era of this history.

A material addition to knowledge of typhus fever came from epidemiologic studies in southeastern United States, where Maxcy (1926) demonstrated a concentration of the disease in cities and towns, and suggested the rat as a reservoir of infection and an ectoparasite of rats as the vector. Two varieties of typhus fever eventually were differentiated, murine and classical louse-borne typhus. Zinsser (1934) recognized Brill's disease as recurrent louse-borne typhus, and this knowledge has been extended by Murray and Snyder (1951). Q fever, once looked upon as a disease indigenous to Australia, was found in western United States (Davis and Cox, 1938) (Dyer, 1939), at first presumably as a sporadic infection of man but soon demonstrated as a disease of cattle, and hence of persons exposed through the livestock and dairy industries.

A natural consequence of World War II was a renewed interest in louse-borne typhus (Am. Assn. Adv. Sci., 1950) and in a disease new to Americans, scrub typhus (Blake et al., 1945) of the orient or tsutsugamushi disease. The United States of America

Typhus Commission made significant contributions in both fields. Finally, a new rickettsial disease was discovered (Greenberg et al., 1947), primarily through simple field observations that were quickly confirmed through laboratory identification of the agent, that of rickettsialpox (Huebner, Stamps and Armstrong, 1946). A distribution of the disease beyond the originally defined limits in New York City is being established (Pike, Cohen, and Murray, 1950).

Bacterial Diseases.—Knowledge of the bacteria had reached an earlier stage of perfection than that for the viruses and rickettsiae. Consequently fewer fundamental developments were to be expected in recent years.

When scarlet fever was established as a streptococcal disease (Dick and Dick, 1924), (Dochez and Sherman, 1924), field and laboratory studies soon brought out a common relationship between that disease, streptococcal sore throat, erysipelas, much of puerperal sepsis, and a variety of other pyogenic infections. The principle was thereby strengthened, that clearly distinguishable clinical entities may in fact constitute a single epidemiologic entity, with common measures applicable in prevention and control. The principle, of course, is not new; it was long ago demonstrated in pneumonic and bubonic plague.

A second general principle was established through recognition that a variety of infectious agents are characterized by biologic types which commonly breed true in the course of an epidemic. Before 1920, the pneumococci had been divided into three specific types, and a fourth having no homogeneity and known to contain serologically different strains. The means for an improved classification were perfected (Heidelberger and Avery, 1923), with at least 75 types now recognized, many with more or less regularly occurring and individual epidemiological characteristics. The hemolytic streptococci were separated into 12 groups (Lancefield, 1928), with Group A found to be the common pathogen of man. Group A streptococci were subdivided into some 40 serological types (Lancefield, 1933) with demonstrated differences in geographical distribution and pathogenicity. A method of separating types of typhoid bacilli through action of bacteriophages (Craigie and Yen, 1938) was a Canadian contribution. An improved classification of meningococci led to the important epidemiological demonstration (Branham, 1940) that most epidemics of the United States were due to Group I.

Similar studies have had the objective, not of typing strains within a species but of separating species within closely related groups of pathogenic agents. Perhaps the greatest precision in differentiating antigenic patterns was in respect to salmonella, with American workers (Edwards and Rettger, 1927) contributing to the extensive information originating in Britain and Denmark. Relationships among the dysentery bacilli were better defined. As a result of the work of Evans (1918), the biologic varieties of brucella attained new significance and permitted an improved epidemiological approach. The viruses were also concerned, through recognition of a variety of infectious agents in the arthropod-borne encephalitides and the influenzas.

The main incentive in both lines of investigation was to acquire information permitting improved measures for active immunization and specific biological therapy. Some progress was made in the first endeavor, but the introduction of the sulfonamides and of antibiotic therapy largely ended interest in the second objective. For many diseases, however, the separation of types and related species has provided the means for a more precise and intelligent field practice.

The intestinal infections of bacterial origin have been much studied, for despite adequate knowledge of such major conditions as typhoid fever and cholera, the pathogenic agents responsible for the diarrheas and the dysenteries are still an enigma. Active investigations by Hardy (1948) and by Watt (1948) and others have marked progress in understanding.

Protozoal Diseases.—A common saying among epidemiologists is that to know malaria is to understand the basic principles of epidemiology. For that opinion, there is justification. No disease gives better illustration of theory turned to practice. Few diseases include so many features of the total composite that enters into multiple causation. Field method is highly developed, whether the objective is research or control. If the criterion is practical accomplishment, the disease is now so uncommon in the United States that case study instead of the enumeration of deaths has the attention of epidemiologists. Reported cases of malaria in 1949 in continental United States were 4,241 (Andrews, Quinby, and Langmuir, 1950). Primary indigenous infections, especially if confirmed by identification of the parasite, were a small fraction of that number. Conditions may be compared with those of 1900, when deaths alone numbered 2,434 and cases ran into the hundreds of thousands.

Fungus Diseases.—Of known infectious agents, the fungi are not particularly important as causes of disease in man, but one of them, coccidioidomycosis, has a place in this review if for no other reason than that what is known epidemiologically is almost wholly of American origin (Smith, 1940). Histoplasmosis is another actively investigated disease, both in field (Furcolow, High, and Allen, 1946) and laboratory (Emmons, Olson, and Eldridge, 1945). The fungi themselves have had the attention of a group of workers (Conant et al., 1944).

General.—One final principle relates to the introduction of chemotherapeutic measures and antibiotic therapy. These measures have had a profound effect on the epidemiological behavior of infections. Fatality and mortality rates for many diseases have been remarkably reduced. Morbidity has been affected in a number of instances through use of these products in prevention as distinguished from therapy, but another influence on morbidity is not so universally appreciated. A new epidemiologic principle has indeed developed. Therapeutic use of these substances often so shortens the period of communicability that fewer reservoirs of infection, sick persons, are present in a community at a given time. The community dosage is, therefore, less, and the potentiality of transmission limited. The practical significance is evident in the recent edition of *Control of Communicable Diseases in Man* (Am. Pub. Health Assn., 1950), where the principle is judged applicable to thirty-nine of eight-two listed diseases.

The advances in knowledge of mass disease just recorded are ample proof that progress in epidemiology is closely related to progress in microbiology. The theory of multiple causation carries no implication of a lesser emphasis on the agent in mass disease, but recognizes two other coordinate elements in causation, one of which, the host, now has our attention.

Host Factor

The significance of latent infection and latent immunization has come to full realization in this modern era, and also an improved ability to measure and evaluate these phenomena. Technical procedure suited to wide scale use of serological methods has led to a new kind of field method, serological epidemiology. An early use was in estimating antitoxin content of the blood in diphtheria. Neutralization tests for poliomyelitis were applied in field practice. The mouse protection test in yellow fever (Sawyer and Lloyd, 1931) illustrates the widest use of these methods, and studies of the past history of poliomyelitis among Eskimos (Paul and Riordan, 1950) are a recent application.

Immunological tests such as the tuberculin reaction, the skin test for mumps, those for scarlet fever, diphtheria, and a number of others have proved practical means for sorting out susceptible and immune individuals in the field.

The technics of pathologic anatomy have also been turned to field survey use, with viscerotome specimens of the liver (Soper, Rickard, and Crawford, 1934) providing material for identification of deaths from yellow fever and leishmaniasis in South America and Africa.

A further contribution, not always appreciated, is the increased exactness conferred upon field data through use of a variety of serological procedures in clinical diagnosis.

The improved regard for the host factor in causation of mass disease reflected also on those inherent factors generally classed as autarcesis. Inherent insusceptibility is a good deal more than genetically determined characteristics, important as they are in the species, racial, individual, and constitutional differences manifest in many diseases.

Anatomical considerations came to be appreciated as the main factor in such situations as the disproportionately high fatality of laryngeal diphtheria among infants under one year, with the reason a smaller trachea and the likelihood of suffocation, and not a greater activity of diphtheria toxin. Tissue injury incident to tonsillectomy (Aycock, 1942) and parenteral injections (Anderson and Skaar, 1951) were recognized as determining factors in the frequency of paralysis in poliomyelitis infections.

Physiological variations of the host clearly act in determining health and disease. Some of the sex differences in poliomyelitis have been related to pregnancy (Aycock, 1941) and menstruation (Weinstein, Aycock, and Feemster, 1951). Seasonal differences in susceptibility to experimental syphilis of rabbits (Pearce, 1938) and mumps in monkeys (Johnson and Goodpasture, 1930) are known, and they are not due to changes in the infectious agent. Endocrine characteristics and hormonal imbalance (Dempsey, 1951) receive current attention. These innate factors of the host, like the specific response of immunity, are sometimes temporary and again permanent.

Webster (1946) in his experimental studies of mouse populations did much to demonstrate genetic relationships. Schneider (1951) has investigated physiological and metabolic considerations related to nutrition, with much remaining to be done in measuring added environmental effect on the host.

The potentialities of clinical study and field methods in better understanding of these inherent factors in resistance are far from exhausted. From a laboratory standpoint, the time would appear at hand when the immunologist must yield to the biochemist in the next basic advance of knowledge about resistance to disease.

Environment

An understanding of environment as an epidemiological principle requires the triphasic concept of a physical, a biological, and a social environment.

Physical Environment.—An environmental sanitation and a geography of disease were direct outgrowths of early interest in physical features of the environment. Work in historical and geographical pathology lapsed unwarrantedly with the coming of bacteriology, to be revived under pressure of necessity during World War II. This sort of information was appreciated as essential to military operations. Under army auspices, a comprehensive geography of disease was brought together under the title *Global Epidemiology* (Simmons et al., 1944). The stimulus continues (Light, 1944). World maps of poliomyelitis and cholera are among recent contributions (May, 1950) with the aim to present one disease as a world problem in substitution for the more usual effort centered on one region and all its diseases.

Biological Environment.—Epidemiologic interest in the biologic environment was early concerned with those diseases which attack both man and animal. The circumstances by which an infectious agent passed from animal to man were demonstrated to be of varied nature. Sometimes transfer was direct from animal to man but with a blind ending, for further passage within a human population did not occur. Sometimes both man and animal were infected from a third source. Sometimes the agency of an arthropod vector was required. The separation of these tangled relationships has been a fascinating part of epidemiology, of which the ecology of plague (Meyer, 1942) is a good illustration. Theobald Smith (1934) developed basic concepts through his studies on parasitism and disease. Karl Meyer (1948) recently has brought together existing facts from his own and other experience to give a critical interpretation of homologous and heterologous chains of infection.

Much practical value to man has arisen from studies on brucellosis (Am. Assn. Adv. Sci., 1950), leptospirosis (Meyer, Stuart-Anderson, and Eddie, 1939), tularemia (Simpson, 1929) and many others. These interests have extended to such problems as jungle yellow fever and a search for the hidden reservoir of rabies. Epidemiologists with a primary concern of human disease have been increasingly drawn to this wider phase of the ecologic universe, for the simple reason that a knowledge of animal disease has many times proved essential to understanding of disease in man.

Arthropod-borne infections are now recognized as one of the five great classes among communicable diseases, as judged by mode of transmission. Significant contributions crowded the early part of the twentieth century and in the course of the past thirty years they have multiplied many times. Because entomologists have had a natural part in these studies, progress has been along broad biologic lines, and ecologically flavored. Because of the nature and magnitude of the problems as mass diseases of man, epidemiologists commonly have been concerned with a single disease or a group of diseases. Hackett (1937), Boyd (1949) and Russell (1946) have thus worked with malaria, Sawyer (1937) and Soper (1937) with yellow fever, and Hammon (1948) with the arthropod-borne encephalitides. As knowledge accumulated about arthropods, empiric facts about causation, once attributed to climate, sun, atmosphere and soil were seen in a truer perspective as influences that act through the effect they have on arthropod vectors.

The discovery within the past decade of DDT and related compounds was not only the greatest single event among arthropod-borne diseases, but ranks with the antibiotics and chemotherapy among outstanding advances of this whole modern period. Malaria has been reduced in some parts of the world to limits judged improbable a decade ago. Principle in the epidemic control of plague (Gordon and Knies, 1947) has turned from attack on the rat to the destruction of fleas. Typhus fever (Am. Assn. Adv. Sci., 1950) in the last great war was no problem at all, compared with previous experience. The effect has been more than on these great epidemic diseases; it has indeed extended to the whole solid bulk of endemic, insect-borne infection.

Social Environment.—The report of a developing knowledge on social factors as an influence on mass disease is not so satisfying; but to have this field recognized at long last as a part of epidemiology is no mean accomplishment. Some tangible progress has been made, with population pressures (Milbank Memorial Fund, 1950), housing (Am. Pub. Health Assn., 1950), social motivations (N. Y. Acad. Med., 1949), and the provisions of a satisfactory program for medical care (Goldmann and Leavell, 1951) among subjects having had attention in recent times. The chief limiting factor in transferring conceptual scheme to practice was a lack of adequate data by which to appraise events. That deficiency would seem to have had its origin, first in an unsatisfactory definition of terms understandable alike to biologist and social scientist, and second in a field method failing of facts that could be counted and measured. The social scientist warrants a more active place on the epidemiologic team. A cheering example of progress is to be had in the modern approach to tuberculosis (Perkins, 1950). Well-controlled studies, such as those of Jean Downes (1950) on the effect of vitamin supplementation among household contacts to tuberculosis, are needed.

Operational Activities

Public health deals with groups of people, and epidemiology is the study of disease behavior as manifested by groups. For this reason epidemiology is accepted as a basic science of public health. It occupies no exclusive position, for all of the sciences of preventive medicine come into play, and other disciplines are of greater importance in the control and management of community disease. It is basic in the sense that it is the point of departure, the means by which mass disease is recognized and appraised. It is perhaps best understood as the counterpart of diagnosis in clinical medicine (Gordon, 1950). As such, epidemiology is an operational discipline and the extent of its application progressively enlarges.

Health Departments

Epidemiological investigations were a part of health department practice from the time when health departments were established, but Minnesota was the first state officially to appoint an epidemiologist, H. W. Hill in 1909. Only a few states, in 1920, had divisions of epidemiology supplying an acceptable quality of service (Ferrell, 1942), and the number was not great in 1930. Most states now have creditable divisions of epidemiology, and so have the larger cities. Organizational plans vary widely. One state may combine epidemiology and the public health laboratory in a single division. Another may break up the division of epidemiology into separate organizations responsible for a specific disease, as tuberculosis, pneumonia, malaria, or the venereal diseases. A division of disease control, including such divergent activities as cancer, diabetes, and accidental injuries along with the communicable diseases, is often found in present-day practice. In local agencies, a trained epidemiologist often combines that work with other duties; and in the basic county unit, the health officer is also the epidemiologist. At all levels, epidemiologic methods and concepts have permeated the nation's public health structure.

One of the outstanding applications of the epidemiologic method is to guide and evaluate administrative practice, with the Committee on Evaluation of Administrative Practices of the American Public Health Association having had no small part in stimulus to that use. The primary aim is to determine the essential causes active in a given situation so that a program for control and the forces of public health education may be specifically directed, avoiding dissipation of effort on inconsequential objectives. The second requirement is to determine by designed experiment under field conditions the actual effectiveness of the program instituted. The secondary attack rate, as developed by Chapin and enlarged by Frost (1938) has become classical procedure. Illustrative studies in evaluation of administrative practice by epidemiological means are to be found in reports on the effect of oiled floors and bedding on the incidence of respiratory disease (The Commission on Respiratory Diseases, 1946), on pertussis vaccine (Bell, 1948) in protection of children against whooping cough, and on the value of chemoprophylaxis in the control of meningococcal infections (Phair and Schoenbach, 1944).

Military Epidemiology

Epidemiology has become as thoroughly incorporated in the practice of military preventive medicine (Gordon, 1948) as in civilian public health. Over-all direction of epidemiologic activities is in the Preventive Medicine Service of the Surgeon General. All headquarters, from theater of operations to the field army, include an epidemiologist in tables of organization. The duties of medical inspectors of corps and divisions are primarily in preventive medicine and epidemiology.

An advisory and investigative organization known as the Board for the Investigation and Control of Influenza and other Epidemic Diseases in the Army was formed (Army Medical Bulletin, 1942) to meet the emergency needs of World War II. The extent of its contributions are seen in a series of three volumes of collected reports (Army Epidemiological Board, 1941-1945). The work of the board was such that a permanent organization was effected at the close of the war as the Armed Forces Epidemiological Board, with special commissions to deal with selected diseases. Although primarily concerned with communicable diseases, the scope of interests includes traumatic injuries, particularly accidents, and the epidemiology of mental disorder.

The United States of America Typhus Commission (Bayne-Jones, 1947) functioned during the war as an independent special commission, primarily investigational, but providing consultation and occasionally operational aid in situations relating to rickettsial disease.

International Interests

An international view of disease processes, with the world the selected universe, was a natural outgrowth of the comparative method of epidemiological study. Material variations in the character and behavior of a disease according to time and place of occurrence were apparent at an early date. Although some situations strongly favor greater prevalence, few diseases are restricted to a single set of environmental circumstances or to a particular kind of people. Communicable disease tends to spread from country to country, and hence the need for knowledge of international incidence. The modern technology of transport and travel has increased the difficulties, to the extent that an international viewpoint is more or less essential to adequate control of communicable disease in a limited region.

The Indian Plague Commission (Reports on Plague Investigations in India, 1906) was an early recognition of this principle. Other special purpose commissions so proved their usefulness that need became apparent for a continuing organization, supported by the society of nations. The Office International d'Hygiène Publique was a start (1909). The League of Nations saw perhaps its greatest accomplishment in the Health Section, where its epidemiological reports (League of Nations, 1922) and special studies marked clear progress in an international attitude toward epidemiology. After a lapse during the recent war years, activities were revived through an emergency organization known as UNRRA (United Nations Relief and Rehabilitation Association, 1945).

With the establishment of the World Health Organization, international epidemiological activities (World Health Organization, 1947) have reached a high level. The central office in Geneva is a source of medical intelligence. Branch offices have been established in several parts of the world, that for the American hemisphere being incorporated in the Pan American Sanitary Bureau. Expert commissions study specific diseases. International commissions, in which American epidemiologists take part, have served in a special purpose capacity from time to time in a number of countries. World centers have been established for the study of specific diseases such as influenza, salmonella infections, and brucellosis in appreciation that the epidemiology of any disease under modern conditions is only to be understood through an international approach. The World Center for Influenza, for example, has its headquarters in London, with branches in Australia, America, and a number of European countries. It collects and distributes information on the world occurrence of the disease, collects strains of virus and studies their antigenic nature, in search of information of new strains and knowledge of how they pass from one country to another.

Epidemiology in the Tropics

The concept of tropical medicine has changed from that of a peculiar group of diseases persisting in peculiar parts of the world to an appreciation that tropical medicine is general medicine, and that few truly tropical diseases exist. For various reasons, including a favorable climate or a climate not unfavorable, a goodly number of infectious processes have an undue frequency and exhibit an individual behavior in the tropics. Most of them, however, extend widely into subtropical regions and not infrequently into temperate areas.

A number of events in recent years have turned American epidemiology and American epidemiologists to more serious consideration of this previously unfamiliar field. The recent world war took American soldiers to many parts of the world, and for the first time to a full scale war in the tropics. The expanding political influences that forced this country into a world position were another consideration. Technical changes in trade and traffic are such that the world tends rapidly to become a single epidemiologic universe.

By reason of the growing concept of tropical medicine just stated, an epidemiologic interest in almost any disease is seen to have a relation to tropical problems. To this extent Americans were concerned with the epidemiology of tropical diseases, but practical responsibility was limited for many years to the Panama Canal Zone and Hawaii. A more active participation through field work in tropical areas followed the Spanish American War, when this country took on obligations for populations of the Philippines, Puerto Rico, and some other areas. Federal and military workers acquired experience in operational procedures in tropical countries and made field investigations of bacillary dysentery (Flexner, 1900), dengue fever (Simmons, 1931), and a variety of other diseases. The main feature of a developing American interest in tropical epidemiology, especially during the early part of this period 1920-1950, was a series of studies by staff members of the International Health Division of the Rockefeller Foundation in a number of countries and on a variety of diseases, yellow fever, hookworm disease, schistosomiasis, malaria and others.

As a direct result of military operations after 1940, tropical medicine and tropical epidemiology took on new significance. Facilities of the armed forces were enlarged and new workers drawn to the field. Commissions undertook study of special problems, and operational needs were met.

A satisfying aftermath of this emergency activity is the extent to which interest has continued. The American Society of Tropical Medicine has taken on new life. The armed forces continue work in the field; the Navy, with a permanent epidemiological unit in Cairo (Shaw, 1950), the Army with basic studies at the Army Medical Service Graduate School and such field activities as scrub typhus (Philip, Traub, and Smadel, 1949) and typhoid fever in Malaya. Formal courses of instruction in tropical medicine, with emphasis on epidemiology, have been organized in a number of schools of public health; and the preventive medicine courses of medical schools give these interests increasing attention. Most promising of all is the research activity in many centers, by epidemiologists and by workers in allied disciplines, notably those of nutrition, biochemistry, and physiology.

The principal advances in tropical medicine have been in clinical knowledge of the diseases there present, of the agents responsible and of the vectors involved. These are to be recognized as parts of a broader problem. An improved understanding of disease in the tropics would seem to require added stress on the study of these conditions as mass phenomena of disease, in respect to herd reactions, having as an objective that epidemiologic interpretation so largely accomplished for diseases of temperate regions. The pattern has been set by studies on malaria and yellow fever.

Progress of Epidemiology as a Profession

Epidemiology has been practiced for a long time (Winslow, 1943). If the formation of the London Epidemiological Society in 1850 is taken as a determining date, it has existed as a recognized scientific discipline for at least 100 years (Transactions Epidemiological Society, London, 1855). Its development into an independent profession, however, is almost within the present historical period, 1920-1950. In America, epidemiology as a profession may well be dated from 1909, for in that year Hill became the first duly appointed epidemiologist in a health department, and the first department of preventive medicine in a medical school was founded at Harvard, where Milton J. Rosenau based his conception of preventive medicine on epidemiology as the fundamental discipline.

Plans incident to the founding of the Johns Hopkins School of Hygiene and Public Health made provision for a chair of epidemiology. In 1921, Wade Hampton Frost became the first professor of epidemiology in America. He remains the first among all who have followed, for no one has done more to further epidemiology as a scientific discipline. As new schools of public health were founded, with ten now existing in the United States and one in Canada, they were organized around a central core of disciplines, usually including sanitary engineering, biostatistics, and public health practice, and each with a professor of epidemiology.

The increasing academic interest in epidemiology and the growing numbers giving attention to operational epidemiology in official health departments resulted in the organization of the American Epidemiological Society in November, 1927. Haven Emerson and Edward S. Godfrey, Jr., were primarily instrumental in bringing this about. Charles V. Chapin served as the first president, and the twenty-fifth year of meetings has just passed. Two years later, in 1929, the American Public Health Association established an epidemiological section with seven fellows and one member on the original rolls. Don M. Griswold was the first chairman of the section, Godfrey was vice-chairman, and Haven Emerson the secretary. The roster of members has increased substantially each year, until at the present time, in 1950, there are 166 fellows and 480 members of the section, which is seventh among the 13 sections of the Association.

These two societies have contributed importantly to American epidemiology. The interests of the American Epidemiologic Society are primarily those of the learned society, concerned with the establishment of principle, the development of theory, and the evaluation of progress; and devoting attention at the annual meetings, more to work in progress than to completed studies. The Epidemiology Section of the American Public Health Association serves the broader purpose of a forum for presentation of reports of work done and methods developed. It has interest in plans for epidemiological services in state and local health organizations, for the collection and utilization of data on morbidity and mortality, for the study of epidemic and endemic disease, and for the selection and training of personnel for these services. The preparation of the authoritative manual on *The Control of Communicable Diseases in Man*, now one of the most widely used medical books in America, is an outstanding accomplishment of the Association, in which members of the section have taken an important and continuing part.

About 1915, the United States Public Health Service began enlarging its epidemiological activities; and no small part of the progress in epidemiology since then has had its origin in that leadership. Allen W. Freeman was the first epidemiologist appointed in the service, in March of 1915. The Hygienic Laboratory, originally established in 1902, progressively increased its field activities and eventually grew into the National Institutes of Health. Conceived as a center for laboratory research, the institution has always held to the policy of extending observations to the field. Branch laboratories have been established to study a number of diseases in areas in which they prevail, notably the Rocky Mountain Spotted Fever Laboratory in Montana and the Plague Laboratory in California. Groups of workers from the central institute commonly set up headquarters in the field for emergency or continued study of particular situations. Through a system of grants-in-aid, administered by commissions associated with the Institutes of Health, funds are provided in support of epidemiologic studies in universities, in official health departments, and in voluntary health organizations.

To facilitate field activities, the Public Health Service in 1946 established a Communicable Disease Center in Atlanta, Georgia, this being an outgrowth of a wartime organization for epidemiologic service in regions about military camps. Based on strong divisions for laboratory and field study, the mission of the Communicable Disease Center is to provide consultation and aid to state and local health services. It functions through a central organization and through field stations in various parts of the country. Although conceived as a service organization, with the additional aim to train personnel of state and local health departments, an inevitable result of its activities has been a broad contribution to new knowledge. A further gain becomes increasingly apparent in the substantial effect the work of the Center is having on the quality of epidemiologic practice at state and local level.

The practice of epidemiology in the United States would scarcely be what it is today without the aid and encouragement that have come from the great voluntary health organizations which are so much a part of the American scheme. Of those with general interests, the work of the Rockefeller Foundation requires no comment beyond that already made. The Milbank Memorial Fund has pioneered epidemiological exploration in a variety of fields, notably in tuberculosis, nutrition, and mental disorder; and in population pressures as they affect all mass disease. The Commonwealth Fund has had a continuing concern in the epidemiologic method as it relates to public health practice and the evaluation of programs for control. The W. K. Kellogg Foundation has sponsored numerous field studies, and taken more than usual interest in the education of field workers. The numerous voluntary health organizations with interests limited to a single disease or group of diseases, almost without exception have included epidemiologic investigation in their programs; some, such as the Natonal Foundation for Infantile Paralysis, notably so. National societies fostering epidemiologic study include among others those concerned with heart disease, cancer, diabetes, tuberculosis, multiple sclerosis, and aid of crippled children. The part taken by the voluntary health organizations has been in a variety of directions. To a limited extent, studies have been conducted by the organization itself. To a greater extent, interest has had the form of sponsoring short institutes for discussion and analysis of problems, and through support of investigations by individuals and by staffs of official health agencies and educational institutions.

THE CHANGING CHARACTER OF MASS DISEASE PROBLEMS

The mass disease problems of communities of people have altered notably within a century. The reasons are many. They relate both to man as an organism and to the environment in which he lives. Some mass diseases now have far less significance; others have come from an inconsequential place to rank among the leading causes of death or as major factors in lost efficiency or disabling illness. What has happened, however, is more than a matter of numbers of persons affected. In many instances the nature and character of a mass disease have changed. Less often new problems have been introduced by reason of a shifting ecological state. The communicable diseases provide the best illustration of these several considerations, principally because they have been studied most, and because custom has long marked the group as the type of mass disease problem.

Communicable Diseases

Comparing present conditions with those that existed 100 years ago, the changes that have occurred among the communicable diseases are so great as to simulate another world. Intestinal infections are far less frequent. Diseases transmitted through discharges of the upper respiratory tract are relatively more important among infections in general. The situation is less definite for diseases spread by direct contact, although these conditions likewise tend to become of greater moment as agglomeration of peoples becomes more pronounced; the venereal diseases, as representative of the class, are about as frequent as ever. An improved control of arthropod-borne disease has been an outstanding accomplishment of recent years. Of diseases of man originating from animals, more has been done about infections associated with domestic animals than where wild animals are the reservoir. No reason exists for believing that the actual frequency of diseases of animal origin has increased, but relatively they become more important among classes of communicable disease because of the greater numbers identified, and the fewer arising from other sources.

One or other of two general means is useful in judging quantitatively the changes that have taken place in the frequency of communicable disease. The first is through comparing computed rates of incidence in terms of units of population. The second is through examining the relative standing of infections among mass diseases as causes of death.

In 1900, the ten leading causes of death in the United States included five infectious diseases; the current list has only two. First place in 1900 was occupied by an infectious disease, tuberculosis; by 1948 the highest rank of a communicable process was seventh, for pneumonia and influenza, and tuberculosis was eighth. The community problems of the present, as measured in terms of death, are resident in diseases not communicable nor caused by a specific infectious agent. They include heart disease, the neoplasms, and diabetes; and also mass injuries as distinguished from mass disease. Much the same judgment holds when the criteria are defect and disability. Although no disease has supplanted the common cold as a disabling illness, the nutritional deficiencies and the neuropsychiatric disorders have high rank.

The main direction of effort in epidemiology is still toward communicable diseases. It becomes increasingly evident, however, that a limitation of activities to the infections is no longer warranted. That conviction is supported to the extent that it may be accepted as principle, applying with little reservation to the countries of North America and western Europe. It is in line with the altered conditions of the new world. There is to be no misunderstanding that this view implies any slackening of effort against such communicable diseases as tuberculosis and the pneumonias, which are still among the major problems of public health. Furthermore, the gains that have brought other diseases still lower on the scale must be held. For many countries the communicable diseases will continue as the first consideration, and for a long time. They will have strong consideration in America, with a secondary reason for their study being the favorable means they provide for gaining familiarity with the epidemiologic method. The reasonable approach to the broader and less well explored fields of mass disease is through expansion and transfer of that method.

Noncommunicable Organic Disease

Heart disease now ranks as the first cause of death in the United States; and deaths from cancer, from circulatory disturbances, from metabolic diseases, and degenerative processes are well up on the list. A direct relation is seen with the altered social and economic conditions of the present century. Many of the changes have been brought about by the advancing age of the American population. With fewer deaths from communicable disease, people now live longer; and long enough to acquire conditions which are largely limited to older people.

The practical result of this shifting situation is an established and increasing trend among public health workers to accord greater emphasis to diseases characteristic of old age. This is a reasonable attitude, as has been demonstrated. However, a satisfactory perspective and a balanced judgment are necessary in the newly developed enthusiasm about geriatrics. The health of children is still the important consideration among public health problems, admittedly not because of the single relation to communicable disease, but because of disorders associated with nutrition, growth, development, and the varied psychiatric disturbances. The child has a life expectancy of many years; that of the older group is brief. The greater profit in years of healthful living is alone sufficient reason for greater stress on the mass diseases of childhood. The kind of years that are gained also has significance; for the child, these are years of productive and creative effort; for the older person they are likely to be not only few but relatively unproductive.

In recent years, epidemiological methods have been applied in American practice to dental fluorosis (Black and McKay, 1916) and dental caries (Dean, 1938), to cancer (Levin, 1948) and to multiple sclerosis (Kurland and Moriyama, 1951), to diseases of the heart (Dawber, Meadors, and Moore, 1951) and to diabetes (Wilkerson and Krall, 1947), and even to such unusual fields as the congenital anomalies (Ingalls and Gordon, 1947) and atmospheric pollution (Schrenk et al., 1949). The list is by no means inclusive.

Mental Disorder

Of all mass health problems of communities, more interest has been given to organic disease than to functional disturbances (Wearn, 1947). A number of reasons account for this attitude. There is greater ease of recognition, a more ready establishment of cause, and a greater availability of methods for measuring both cause and effect. It is just being appreciated that mental disorders, the problems of addiction to alcohol and drugs, and the social diseases concerned with occupation, recreation, and the intellectual pursuits of man, also constitute group as well as individual problems. As a field in epidemiology these mass diseases of emotional and mental origin have scarcely been touched. There is indication of a developing activity (Milbank Memorial Fund, 1950).

Injuries

Some fifty years ago the duties of a physician came to be understood as something more than the care of the sick and the injured. The obligations of the doctor were defined as "first, to prevent disease; if that is not possible, to cure; and if that is impossible, to alleviate." As the new concept of prevention developed, it was applied almost wholly to disease, to the sick. The injured were largely forgotten until the recently aroused interest in the civilian problem of accidents, and in such military conditions as trench foot, battle casualities, and the ordinary injuries of military life. Collectively, these problems constitute an epidemiology of trauma.

Accidents of all forms, as judged by data of 1948, rank fourth among causes of death in the United States. As health problems of communities of people, the traumatic injuries that occur through accident can be demonstrated to conform to the same biologic laws as do those of disease (Gordon, 1949). They are amenable to the same epidemiologic approach and what is less well appreciated, they are preventable and controllable. Instead of something set apart from disease and scarcely to be considered within the scope of preventive medicine, injuries are as much a public health problem as measles.

CURRENT DIRECTION OF EPIDEMIOLOGIC INTERESTS

A wide range of pathologic conditions is included within modern ideas of mass or community disease. The approach to solution of problems concerned with mass disease, as typified by the communicable diseases, has been through epidemiology, a biologic discipline concerned with disease as it affects groups of people. Medicine and public health would thus appear called upon to alter existing interpretations of the field of usefulness of the epidemiologic method. A limitation to the communicable diseases is no longer warranted by present-day conditions. That concept depends upon the assumption that all mass diseases and injuries conform to the same biologic laws of ecology as do communicable processes. It is believed they do.

If an etiologic interpretation of disease and injury is the basis of modern medical practice, and it surely is, then the agents that give rise to the many pathological conditions must be variously viable and nonviable, sometimes transmissible and sometimes not. If morbid conditions of man are the result of a reaction between the human host and his environment, then all disease conditions can be interpreted in terms of three principal factors. The first is the agent, either an inanimate substance or a living thing, that directly gives rise to the condition. The second is the host, the organism injured or affected; and man of all living things is the most important host. The third factor is the environment in which host and agent exist, an environment which has much to do with determining the qualities and activities of both, and additionally has a strong influence on the nature and effectiveness of the interaction that takes place between the two. Thus looked upon, disease and injury, and also the physiologic state, are interpreted as ecologic phenomena and amenable in their group manifestations to the methods of epidemiologic analysis. Epidemiology is seen as a biologic discipline applicable to all disease where groups of persons or living things are involved, to include both plant and animal.

The development of new knowledge or the introduction of new conditions commonly calls for a change in method or a shift in emphasis. The evidence is of a world that tends to become one epidemiologic universe, that is experiencing a changing character of population and an altered social and economic environment. The result is a change in values among mass disease problems. To meet its obligations to preventive medicine and public health, epidemiology is called upon to broaden its interests. As expressed by Dr. Joseph Mountin, "it is high time that epidemiologists escaped their Broad Street pump fixation." The reference of course is to the classical studies of Snow on cholera, where the foundation was laid for field method in epidemiology and from which developed the established association of epidemiology and communicable disease. The implication in this pungent remark is that restriction to a concern of communicable disease, to the neglect of other pressing problems, is no longer justifiable; that epidemiology is obligated to give more attention to mass problems provided by other diseases.

THE FUTURE IN EPIDEMIOLOGY

In starting to write of the History of American Epidemiology and specifically of the yesterday, today, and tomorrow of the twentieth century since 1920, I entered upon the events of the earlier years with confidence. Time has a way of settling the worth of things. The contributions of today have not had that benefit; differences of opinion exist; and sometimes bias enters. Evaluation was more difficult and sometimes less certain. Personal views and personal interpretations inevitably entered; and as will have become evident, I have attempted no more than to set things down as I see them.

The final part of my task, to speak of the tomorrow, is still more exacting. Whatever authority I may possess is in science rather than as a seer. I can do no better than to outline, in place of the usual summary, what to me appears to be the course that epidemiological activities will take in the foreseeable future. Five general lines seem evident:

As the diagnostic discipline of public health, epidemiology should find increasing usefulness in the definition of health problems, in determining principles to guide programs for control, and in evaluation of accomplishment. The promise of a more scientific and a more statesmanlike public health has a close relationship with operational epidemiology.

With all mass disease and mass injury understood as the resultant of ecologic forces within a prescribed universe, epidemiology should escape its still too common restriction to communicable diseases, to find application in organic diseases of noninfective nature, in mental disorder, and in the problems associated with trauma.

There is good reason to believe that the methods of experimental epidemiology, using colonies of animals, will be expanded to other mass disease than that of infectious origin. A beginning has been made with nutritional disorders. Cancer, poisoning by chemical dusts and vapors, and even emotional and mental disorders may well be approached in like manner.

Through planned investigations and prospective observations, in substitute for the more usual comparative and analytical observations on past events, field studies on human populations have the potentiality of an improved instrument for research. That the classical procedures of epidemiology have not been supplanted by this newer approach, as a source of new knowledge, is evidenced in the recent demonstration of congenital anomalies after German measles, which was as fine an example of field epidemiology in the traditional manner as ever recorded.

An enlarged interest in military epidemiology is seen as an inevitable result of the existing times. There will be need to provide epidemiological service to troops operating in a variety of countries and encountering unfamiliar diseases. The potentialities of a biological warfare will have to be defined. Defensive features presumably rest in application of established epidemiological principles, commonly to infectious agents and diseases that are well known, but with no such limitation assured. The offense in biologic warfare is something else, namely, the attempt to produce rather than to limit disease; and that is epidemiology upside down.

References

Allee, W. C., Park, O., Emerson, A. E., Park, T., and Schmidt, K. P.: Principles of Animal Ecology, Philadelphia, Saunders, 1949.

American Association for the Advancement of Science: The Rickettsial Diseases of Man, Washington, 1948.

American Association for the Advancement of Science: Brucellosis, Washington, 1950.

American Public Health Association: An Appraisal Method for Measuring
    the Quality of Housing: a Yardstick for Health Officers, Housing
    Officials and Planners. Part I. Nature and Uses of the Method,
    1945; Part II. Appraisal of Dwelling Conditions. Director's Man-
    ual; Field Procedures; Office Procedures, 1946; Part III. Appraisal
    of Neighborhood Environment, 1950.
American Public Health Association: The Control of Communicable Dis-
    eases in Man, New York, 1950.
Anderson, G. W., and Skaar, A. E.: Poliomyelitis Occurring After Antigen
    Injections, Pediatrics 7: 741, 1951.
Andrews, J. M., Quinby, G. E., and Langmuir, A. D.: Malaria Eradica-
    tion in the United States, Am. J. Pub. Health 40: 1405, 1950.
Army Epidemiological Board, Collected Reprints, Volumes I-III, 1941-1945.
Army Medical Bulletin No. 64: Board for the Investigation and Control
    of Influenza and Other Epidemic Diseases in the Army, October,
    1942, p. 1.
Aycock, W. L.: A Study of the Significance of Geographic and Seasonal
    Variations in the Incidence of Poliomyelitis, J. Prev. Med. 3: 245,
    1929.
Aycock, W. L.: The Frequency of Poliomyelitis in Pregnancy, New Eng-
    land J. Med. 225: 405, 1941.
Aycock, W. L.: Tonsillectomy and Poliomyelitis; I. Epidemiologic Con-
    siderations, Medicine 21: 65, 1942.
Aycock, W. L.: Seasonal Prevalence as a Principle in Epidemiology, Am.
    J. M. Sc. 209: 395, 1945.
Balfour, M. C.: Some Features of Malaria in Greece and Experience With
    Its Control, Riv. di malariol. 30: 152, 1936.
Bayne-Jones, S.: Reciprocal Effects of the Relationship of Bacteriology and
    Medicine, J. Bact. 21: 61, 1931.
Bayne-Jones, S.: The Control of Typhus Fever, Rhode Island M. J. 30:
    423, 1947.
Bell, J. A.: Pertussis Immunization, J. A. M. A. 137: 1273, 1948.
Bigelow, G. H., and Lombard, H. L.: Cancer and Other Chronic Diseases
    in Massachusetts, Boston, Houghton Mifflin Company, 1933.
Black, G. V., and McKay, F. S.: Mottled Teeth; an Endemic Develop-
    mental Imperfection of the Enamel of the Teeth Heretofore Un-
    known in the Literature of Dentistry, Dental Cosmos 58: 129, 1916.
Blake, F. G., Maxcy, K. F., Sadusk, J. F., Jr., Kohls, G. M., and Bell, E. J.:
    Studies on Tsutsugamushi Disease (Scrub Typhus, Mite-Borne Ty-
    phus) in New Guinea and Adjacent Islands: Epidemiology, Clinical
    Observations and Etiology in the Dobadura Area, Am. J. Hyg. 41:
    243, 1945.
Bohr, N.: On the Notions of Causality and Complementarity, Science 111:
    51, 1950.
Boyd, M. F.: Malariology, Philadelphia, W. B. Saunders Company, 1949.
Branham, S. E.: The Meningococcus (Neisseria intracellularis), Bact.
    Rev., 4: 59, 1940.
Bulletin de l'Office International d'Hygiène Publique, Volume 1, 1909.
Bulloch, W.: The History of Bacteriology, London, Oxford University
    Press, 1938.
Chapin, C. V.: The Sources and Modes of Infection, New York, John
    Wiley & Sons, Inc. 1910.
Chapin, C. V.: The Science of Epidemic Diseases, Scient. Monthly, 26:
    481, 1928.
Clark, E. G., and Turner, T. B.: Studies on Syphilis in the Eastern Health
    District of Baltimore City; Study of Prevalence of Syphilis Based on
    Specific Age Groups of Enumerated Populations, Am. J. Pub. Health
    32: 307, 1942.

Commission on Acute Respiratory Diseases and the Commission on Air-Borne Infections: A Study of the Effect of Oiled Floors and Bedding on the Incidence of Respiratory Diseases in New Recruits, Am. J. Hyg. **43:** 120, 1946.

Conant, N. F., Martin, D. S., Smith, D. T., Baker, R. D., and Callaway, J. L.: Manual of Clinical Mycology, Philadelphia, W. B. Saunders Company, 1944.

Craigie, J., and Yen, C. H.: The Demonstration of Types of B. Typhosus by Means of Preparations of Type II Vi Phage, Canad. J. Pub. Health **29:** 448, 1938.

Dalldorf, G., and Sickles, G. M.: An Unidentified, Filtrable Agent Isolated From the Feces of Children With Paralysis, Science **108:** 61, 1948.

Davis, G. E., and Cox, H. R.: A Filter-Passing Infectious Agent Isolated From Ticks, Pub. Health Rep. **53:** 2259, 1938.

Dawber, T. R., Meadors, G. F., and Moore, F. E.: Epidemiological Approaches to Heart Disease; the Framingham Study, Am. J. Pub. Health **41:** 279, 1951.

Dean, H. T.: Epidemiological Studies of Fluoride Waters and Dental Caries, Federal Security Agency, Public Health Service, Washington, Government Printing Office, 1938.

Dempsey, E. W.: Endocrinology Index, vol. 26-40, p. 90, Ann Arbor, Edwards Bros., Inc., 1951.

Dick, G. F., and Dick, G. H.: A Skin Test for Susceptibility to Scarlet Fever, J. A. M. A. **82:** 265, 1924.

Dingle, J. H., Abernethy, T. J., Badger, G. F., Buddingh, G. J., Feller, A. E., Langmuir, A. D., Ruegsegger, J. M., and Wood, W. B.: Primary Atypical Pneumonia, Etiology Unknown, War Medicine **3:** 223, 1943.

Dochez, A. R., and Sherman, L.: The Significance of Streptococcus Hemolyticus in Scarlet Fever and the Preparation of a Specific Antiscarlatinal Serum by Immunization of the Horse to Streptococcus Hemolyticus-Scarlatinae, J. A. M. A. **82:** 542, 1924.

Downes, J.: An Experiment in the Control of Tuberculosis Among Negroes, New York, Milbank Memorial Fund, 1950.

Dubos, R. J.: Louis Pasteur; Free Lance of Science, Boston, Little, Brown and Company, 1950.

Dyer, R. E.: Similarity of Australian "Q" Fever and a Disease Caused by an Infectious Agent Isolated From Ticks in Montana, Pub. Health Rep. **54:** 1229, 1939.

Edwards, H. R.: Tuberculosis Case Finding: Studies in Mass Surveys, Supp. to Am. Rev. Tuberc. **41:** 3, 1940.

Edwards, P. R., and Rettger, L. F.: The Para-Typhoid B Suipestifer Group of Bacteria, J. Bact. **13:** 73, 1927.

Emerson, H.: Public Health Diagnosis, J. Prev. Med. **1:** 401, 1927.

Emmons, C. W., Olson, B. J., and Eldridge, W. W.: Studies of the Role of Fungi in Pulmonary Disease. I. Cross Reactions of Histoplasmin, Pub. Health Rep. **60:** 1383, 1945.

Enders, J. F.: A Summary of Studies on Immunity in Mumps, Tr. & Stud., Coll. Physicians, Philadelphia, Series 4, **13:** 23, 1945.

Epidemiological Society of London, Transactions of . . ., Vol. I, 1855.

Evans, A. C.: Further Studies on Bacterium Abortus and Related Bacteria. II. A Comparison of Bact. Abortus With Bacteria Bronchisepticus and With the Organism Which Causes Malta Fever, J. Infect. Dis. **22:** 580, 1918.

Ferrell, J. A.: Epidemiology in North America During the Past Twenty Years, Am. J. Pub. Health Supp. Vol. 32, No. 3, 1942.

Finke, L. L.: Versuch einer allgemeinen medizinisch-praktischen Geographie worin der historische Theil der einheimischen Völker-und Staaten-Arzeneykunde vorgetragen wird, Leipzig, Weidmann, 1792-1795.

Flexner, S.: On the Etiology of Tropical Dysentery, Bull. Johns Hopkins Hosp. 11: 231, 1900.

Flexner, S.: Experimental Epidemiology, J. Exper. Med. 36: 9, 1922.

Francis, T., Jr.: A New Type of Virus From Epidemic Influenza, Science 92: 405, 1940.

Frost, W. H.: Epidemiologic Studies of Acute Anterior Poliomyelitis, Hygienic Laboratory Bulletin No. 90, Washington, Government Printing Office, 1913.

Frost, W. H.: Epidemiology, in Nelson Loose Leaf System, Preventive Medicine and Public Health, New York, Thomas Nelson & Sons, 1928, vol. II, p. 163.

Frost, W. H.: Risk of Persons in Familial Contact With Pulmonary Tuberculosis, 23: 426, 1933.

Frost, W. H.: The Familial Aggregation of Infectious Diseases, Am. J. Pub. Health 28: 7, 1938.

Frost, W. H., and Gover, M.: The Incidence and Time Distribution of Common Colds in Several Groups Kept Under Continuous Observation, Pub. Health Rep. 47: 1815, 1932.

Furcolow, M. L., High, R. H., and Allen, M. F.: Some Epidemiological Aspects of Sensitivity to Histoplasmin and Tuberculin, Pub. Health Rep. 61: 1132, 1946.

Garrison, F. H.: The Newer Epidemiology, Mil. Surgeon 53: 1, 1923.

Gauld, R. L.: Epidemiological Field Studies of Infectious Hepatitis in the Mediterranean Theater of Operations, Am. J. Hyg. 43: 248, 1946.

Galdston, I.: The Epidemic Constitution in Historic Perspective, Bull. New York Acad. Med. 18: 606, 1942.

Goldberger, J., Wheeler, G. A., and Sydenstricker, E.: A Study of the Diet of Non-Pellagrous and of Pellagrous Households in Textile Mill Communities in South Carolina in 1916, J. A. M. A. 71: 944, 1918.

Goldmann, F., and Leavell, H. R.: Medical Care for Americans, Ann. Am. Acad. Polit. & Social Sc. 273: 1, January, 1951.

Gordon, J. E.: The Strategic and Tactical Influence of Disease in World War II, Am. J. M. Sc. 215: 311, 1948.

Gordon, J. E.: The Epidemiology of Accidents, Am. J. Pub. Health 39: 504, 1949.

Gordon, J. E.: A History of Preventive Medicine in the European Theater of Operations, United States Army, 1941-1945, Washington, Department of the Army, 1949.

Gordon, J. E.: Epidemiology Old and New, J. Michigan State M. Soc. 49: 194, 1950.

Gordon, J. E., and Augustine, D. L.: Tropical Environment and Communicable Disease, Am. J. M. Sc. 216: 343, 1948.

Gordon, J. E., and Kilham, L.: Ten Years in the Epidemiology of Mumps, Am. J. M. Sc. 218: 338, 1949.

Gordon, J. E., and Knies, P. T.: Flea Versus Rat Control in Human Plague, Am. J. M. Sc. 213: 362, 1947.

Gordon, J. E., and le Riche, H.: The Epidemiologic Method Applied to Nutrition, Am. J. M. Sc. 219: 321, 1950.

Greenberg, M., Pellitteri, O., Klein, I. F., and Huebner, R. J.: Rickettsialpox—a Newly Recognized Rickettsial Disease. II. Clinical Observations, J. A. M. A. 133: 901, 1947.

Graunt, J.: Natural and Political Observations Mentioned in a Following Index and Made Upon the Bills of Mortality, London, Martyn, 1676.

Habel, K.:   (a) Vaccination of Human Beings Against Mumps: Vaccine Administered at the Start of an Epidemic. I. Incidence and Severity of Mumps in Vaccinated and Control Groups. Am. J. Hyg. **54:** 295, 1951.   (b) Vaccination of Human Beings Against Mumps: Vaccine Administered at the Start of an Epidemic. II. Effect of Vaccination Upon the Epidemic, Ibid. **54:** 312, 1951.

Hackett, L. W.:   Malaria in Europe, London, Oxford University Press, 1937.

Haeckel, E.:   Über Entwickelungsgang und Aufgabe der Zoologie, Jenaische Ztschr. f. Med. u. Naturw. **5:** 353, 1870.

Hammon, W. M.:   The Arthropod-Borne Virus Encephalitides, Am. J. Trop. Med. **28:** 515, 1948.

Hardy, A. V., and Watt, J.:   Studies of the Acute Diarrheal Diseases, Pub. Health Rep. **63:** 368, 1948.

Harvard School of Public Health Symposium Volume, Virus and Rickettsial Diseases, Cambridge, Harvard University Press, 1940.

Havens, W. P., Jr.:   Properties of the Etiologic Agent of Infectious Hepatitis, Proc. Soc. Exper. Biol. & Med. **58:** 203, 1945.

Heidelberger, M., and Avery, O. T.:   The Soluble Specific Substance of Pneumococcus, J. Exper. Med. **38:** 73, 1923.

Henle, W., Harris, S., Henle, G., Harris, T. N., Drake, M. E., Margold, F., and Stokes, J., Jr.:   Studies on the Agent of Infectious Hepatitis. I. Propagation of the Agent in Tissue Culture and in the Embryonated Hen's Egg, J. Exper. Med. **92:** 271, 1950.

Hill, H. W.:   The New Public Health, New York, The Macmillan Company, 1922.

Hirsch, A.:   Handbook of Geographical and Historical Pathology, Translated by C. Creighton, London, The New Sydenham Society, 1883-1886.

Huebner, R. J., Stamps, P., and Armstrong, C.:   Rickettsialpox—a Newly Recognized Rickettsial Disease. I. Isolation of the Etiological Agent, Pub. Health Rep. **61:** 1605, 1946.

Ingalls, T. H., and Gordon, J. E.:   Epidemiologic Implications of Developmental Arrests, Am. J. M. Sc. **214:** 322, 1947.

Ipsen, J.:   Attack Rates Among Immigrants to Infected Human Populations, Am. J. Pub. Health **40:** 136, 1950.

Jennings, H. S.:   The Biological Basis of Human Nature, New York, W. W. Norton, 1930.

Johnson, C. D., and Goodpasture, E. W.:   Experimental Immunity to the Virus of Mumps in Monkeys, Am. J. Hyg. **23:** 329, 1936.

Jordan, E. O.:   Epidemic Influenza; a Survey. Chicago, American Medical Association, 1927.

Kircher, A.:   Scrutinium pestis physico-Medicum publico commodo recusum. Graecii, Widmanstad, 1740.

Kurland, L. T., and Moriyama, I. M.:   Certification of Multiple Sclerosis as a Cause of Death, J. A. M. A. **145:** 725, 1951.

Lancefield, R. C.:   The Antigenic Complex of Streptococcus Haemolyticus. I. Demonstration of a Type-Specific Substance in Extracts of Streptococcus Haemolyticus, J. Exper. Med. **47:** 91, 1928.

Lancefield, R. C.:   A Serological Differentiation of Human and Other Groups of Hemolytic Streptococci, J. Exper. Med. **57:** 571, 1933.

League of Nations: Monthly Epidemiological Reports 1-15, 1922, 1936; followed by Weekly Epidemiological Reports to 1940.

Levin, M.:   Some Epidemiological Features of Cancer, Cancer **1:** 489, 1948.

Lewis-Faning, E.:   Report on an Enquiry Into the Aetiological Factors Associated With Rheumatoid Arthritis, Ann. Rheumatic Dis., Supp. to Vol. 9, 1950.

Light, R. U.:   The Progress of Medical Geography, Geog. Rev. **34:** 636, 1944.

MacLeod, C. A.: Primary Atypical Pneumonia, M. Clin. North America 27: 670, 1943.

MacLeod, J.: The Quantitative Method in Biology, Manchester, University of Manchester Press, 1926.

Maxcy, K. F.: Clinical Observations on Endemic Typhus (Brill's Disease) in the United States, Pub. Health Rep. 41: 1213, 1926.

May, J. M.: Medical Geography; Its Methods and Objectives, Geog. Rev. 49: 9, 1950.

Merrell, M., and Reed, L. J.: The Epidemiology of Health, in Social Medicine, Its Derivations and Objectives, New York, The Commonwealth Fund, 1949.

Meyer, K. F., Stuart-Anderson, B., and Eddie, B.: Epidemiology of Leptospirosis, Am. J. Pub. Health 29: 347, 1939.

Meyer, K. F.: The Ecology of Plague, Medicine 21: 143, 1942.

Meyer, K. F.: The Animal Kingdom, a Reservoir of Human Disease, Ann. Int. Med. 33: 326, 1948.

Milam, D. F., and Anderson, R. K.: Nutritional Survey of an Entire Rural County in North Carolina, South M. J. 37: 547, 1944.

Modernization Programs in Relation to Human Resources and Population Problems, New York, Milbank Memorial Fund, 1950.

Milbank Memorial Fund: Epidemiology of Mental Disorder, New York, 1950.

Müller, P. T.: Vorlesungen über allgemeine Epidemiologie, Jena, Fischer, 1914.

Murray, E. S., and Snyder, J. C.: Brill's Disease. II. Etiology, Am. J. Hyg. 53: 22, 1951.

National Foundation for Infantile Paralysis Inc.: Collected Reprints of the Grantees, Vol. I-X, 1939-1949, New York.

Neefe, J. R., Gellis, S. S., and Stokes, J., Jr.: Homologous Serum Hepatitis and Infectious (Epidemic) Hepatitis; Studies in Volunteers Bearing on Immunologic and Other Characteristics of the Etiological Agents, Am. J. Med. 1: 3, 1946.

New York Academy of Medicine: Ecology of Health, New York, The Commonwealth Fund, 1949.

Oliphant, J. W., Gilliam, A. G., and Larson, C. L.: Jaundice Following Administration of Human Serum, Pub. Health Rep. 58: 1233, 1943.

Panum, P. L.: Observations Made During the Epidemic of Measles on the Faroe Islands in the Year 1846, New York, American Public Health Association, 1940.

Pasteur, L.: Oeuvres de . . . réunies par Pasteur Vallery Radot, vols. 1-7, Paris, Masson, 1922-1939.

Paul, J. R., and Riordan, J. R.: Observations on Serological Epidemiology. Antibodies to the Lansing Strain of Poliomyelitis Virus in Sera From Alaskan Eskimos, Am. J. Hyg. 52: 202, 1950.

Pearce, L.: Experimental Syphilis of Oriental Origin; Clinical Reaction in the Rabbit, J. Exper. Med. 67: 443, 1938.

Perkins, J. E.: Tuberculosis in the Light of the New Epidemiology, in Tomorrow's Horizon in Public Health, New York, Public Health Association of New York City, 1950.

Perrott, G. St. J., Tibbits, C., and Britten, R. H.: The National Health Survey; Scope and Method of the Nation-Wide Canvass of Sickness in Relation to Its Social and Economic Setting, Pub. Health Rep. 54: 1663, 1939.

Phair, J. J., and Schoenbach, E. B.: The Dynamics of Meningococcal Infections and the Effect of Chemotherapy, Am. J. Hyg. 40: 318, 1944.

Philip, C. B., Traub, R., and Smadel, J. E.: Chloramphenicol (Chloromycetin) in the Chemoprophylaxis of Scrub Typhus (Tsutsugamushi Disease); I. Epidemiological Observations on Hyperendemic Areas of Scrub Typhus in Malaya, Am. J. Hyg. 5: 63, 1949.

Pike, G., Cohen, S., and Murray, E. S.: Rickettsialpox; Report of a Serologically Proven Case Occurring in a Resident of Boston, Mass., New Eng. J. Med. 243: 913, 1950.

Pope, A. S.: Studies on the Epidemiology of Scarlet Fever, Am. J. Hyg. 6: 389, 1926.

Puffer, R. R., Doull, J. A., Gass, R. S., Murphy, W. J., and Williams, W. C.: Use of the Index Case in the Study of Tuberculosis in Williamson County, Am. J. Pub. Health 32: 601, 1942.

Redi, F.: Experimenta circa generationem insectorum ad nobilissimum virum Carolum Data, Amstelodami, Frisii, 1671.

Reed, L. J.: Panel on Epidemiology, Including Environmental and Occupational Cancer, Proc. Nat. Cancer Conf. 1949, New York, American Cancer Society, 1949.

Reports on Plague Investigations in India, J. Hyg. 6: 422, 1906.

Russell, P. F., West, L. S., and Manwell, R. D.: Practical Malariology, Philadelphia, Saunders, 1946.

Sawyer, W. A.: A History of the Activity of the Rockefeller Foundation in the Investigation and Control of Yellow Fever, Am. J. Trop. Med. 17: 35, 1937.

Sawyer, W. A., and Lloyd, W.: Use of Mice in Tests of Immunity Against Yellow Fever, J. Exper. Med. 54: 533, 1931.

Sawyer, W. A., Meyer, K. F., Eaton, M. D., Bauer, J. H., Putnam, P., and Schwentker, F. F.: Jaundice in Army Personnel in the Western Region of the United States and Its Relation to Vaccination Against Yellow Fever, Am. J. Hyg. 39: 337, 1944; 40: 35, 1944.

Scamman, C. L.: Papers of Charles V. Chapin, Selected by F. P. Gorham, New York, The Commonwealth Fund, 1941.

Schneider, H. A.: Nutrition and Resistance to Infection; the Strategic Situation, Vitamins and Hormones 4: 35, 1946.

Schneider, H. A.: Nutrition and Resistance, Am. J. Trop. Med. 31: 174, 1951.

Schrenk, H. H., Heimann, H., Clayton, G. D., Gafafer, W. M., and Wexler, H.: Air Pollution in Donora, Pa.; Epidemiology of the Unusual Smog Episode of October, 1948, Washington, Federal Security Agency, Public Health Service, 1949.

Schwentker, F. F., Janney, J. H., and Gordon, J. E.: Epidemiology of Scarlet Fever, Am. J. Hyg. 38: 207, 1943.

Shaw, C. C.: Panorama of Naval Medical Research, U. S. Armed Forces M. J., 1: 1199, 1950.

Simmons, J. S.: Dengue Fever, Am. J. Trop. Med. 11: 77, 1931.

Simmons, J. S., Whayne, T. F., Anderson, G. W., and Horack, H. M.: Global Epidemiology, Philadelphia, Lippincott, vol. 1, 1944, Part I: India and the Far East; Part 2: The Pacific Area; vol. 2, 1951, Africa and the Adjacent Islands.

Simpson, W. M.: Tularemia, New York, Hoeber, 1929.

Smillie, W. G.: Observations on the Epidemiology of the Common Cold, New England J. Med. 223: 651, 1940.

Smith, C. E.: Epidemiology of Acute Coccidioidomycosis With Erythema Nodosum; "San Joaquin" or "Valley Fever," Am. J. Pub. Health 30: 600, 1940.

Smith, T.: Parasitism and Disease, Princeton, Princeton University Press, 1934.

Snow, J.: Snow on Cholera, New York, The Commonwealth Fund, 1936.

Soper, F. L.: The Newer Epidemiology of Yellow Fever, Am. J. Pub. Health 27: 1, 1937.

Soper, F. L., Rickard, E. R., and Crawford, P. J.: Routine Post-Mortem Removal of Liver Tissue From Rapidly Fatal Fever Cases For Discovery of Silent Yellow Fever Foci, Am. J. Hyg. 19: 549, 1934.

Soper, F. L., and Wilson, D. B.: Anopheles Gambiae in Brazil, 1930 to 1940, New York, The Rockefeller Foundation, 1943.

Spence, J. C.: Family Studies in Preventive Pediatrics, New England J. Med. 243: 205, 1950.

Stokes, A., Bauer, J. H., and Hudson, N. P.: Transmission of Yellow Fever to Macacus Rhesus, Preliminary Note, J. A. M. A. 90: 253, 1928.

Strode, G. K.: Yellow Fever, New York, McGraw Hill Book Company, Inc., 1951.

Sydenstricker, E.: Hagerstown Morbidity Studies; a Study of Illness in a Typical Population Group, Washington, Government Printing Office, 1930.

United Nations Relief and Rehabilitation Administration, Health Division; Epidemiological Information Bulletin, Vol. I, 1945, and Vol. II, 1946.

Van Beneden, P. J.: Animal Parasites and Messmates, New York, Appleton, 1876.

Vaughan, W. T.: Influenza, an Epidemiologic Study, Am. J. Hyg. Monographic Series No. 1, July, 1921.

Watt, J., and Lindsay, D. R.: Diarrheal Disease Control Studies, Pub. Health Rep. 63: 1319, 1948.

Wearn, J. F.: Functional Disease, J. A. M. A. 134: 1517, 1947.

Webster, L. T.: Experimental Epidemiology, Medicine 25: 77, 1946.

Weinstein, L., Aycock, W. L., and Feemster, R. F.: Relation of Sex, Pregnancy and Menstruation to Susceptibility in Poliomyelitis, New England J. Med. 245: 54, 1951.

Wilder, R. M.: Rickettsial Diseases: Discovery and Conquest, Arch. Path. 49: 479, 1950.

Wilkerson, H. L. C., and Krall, L. P.: Diabetes in a New England Town, J. A. M. A. 135: 309, 1947.

Winslow, C.-E. A.: The Conquest of Epidemic Disease, Princeton, Princeton University Press, 1943.

Winslow, C.-E. A.: Editorial: What Is Epidemiology? Am. J. Pub. Health 38: 852, 1948.

World Health Organization: Epidemiological and Vital Statistics Reports, Vols. 1-4, Geneva, Palais des Nations, 1947-1951.

Zinsser, H.: Varieties of Typhus Virus and the Epidemiology of the American Form of European Typhus Fever (Brill's Disease). Am. J. Hyg. 20: 513, 1934.

Zotta, G.: Études sur le paludisme dans le delta du Danube, Arch. roumaines de path. exper. et de microbiol., 5: 133, 1932.

INDEX OF PERSONS

A

Abbott, A. C., 83, 85
Abbott, S. W., 101
Abel, R., 91
Ackerknecht, E. H., 46
Adami, J. G., 91
Adams, Hugh, 14
Adams, John, 32
Agramonte, A., 88, 90
d'Agramont, Jacme, 21, 22
Albrecht, H., 90
Allee, W. C., 116
Allen, M. F., 142
Allyn, Captain Joseph, 26
Anderson, G. W., 143
Anderson, J. F., 88, 91
Anderson, R. K., 134
Andrews, John B., 82
Andrews, J. M., 141
Armstrong, C., 140
Ashburn, P. M., 88
Augustine, D. L., 116
Avery, O. T., 91, 140
Avicenna, 21
Aycock, W. L., 125, 126, 143

B

Bailey, Richard, 38
Baker, Josephine, 77, 78
Balfour, M. C., 127
Bartlett, Elisha, 32
Bassi, Agostino, 74
Bauer, J. H., 138
Bayne-Jones, S., 115, 148
Beebe, A. L., 90
Bell, J. A., 147
Bentham, Jeremy, 32
Berkeley, Bishop George, 18
Bigelow, G. H., 133
Billings, John Shaw, 79, 80
Black, G. V., 157
Blake, F. G., 139
Blue, Rupert, 90
Boerhaave, Hermann, 27, 28
Bohr, Niels, 120
Bolduan, C. F., 63
Bowditch, Henry P., 81
Boyd, M. F., 59, 127, 145
Boylston, Zabdiel, 13, 19, 20
Branham, S. E., 141
Brill, N. E., 89
Britten, R. H., 133

Brouardel, P., 91
Brown, John, 16, 28, 32
Brown, Walter H., 131
Brownlee, John, 103
Buerger, L., 90
Bulloch, W., 118

C

Cardanus, Hieronymus, 46
Carey, Matthew, 29
Carlisle, R. J., 88
Carroll, J., 88, 90
Carter, Henry R., 97, 98, 99, 103,
   106
Caulfield, Ernest, 13, 14, 15, 16
Celsus, 18
Chadwick, Edwin, 29, 32, 47
Chagas, Carlos, 90
Chapin, Charles V., 88, 95, 96, 97,
   100, 115, 119, 126, 131, 147,
   152
Chickering, H. T., 91
Chowning, W. M., 99
Clark, E. G., 134
Clark, P. F., 91
Clark, Taliaferro, 81
Clot-Bey, Le Dr., 54
Cobden, Richard, 32
Cohen, S., 140
Cole, R., 91
Collins, S. D., 79, 80, 86
Conant, N. F., 142
Conn, H. W., 94
Conradi, H., 90
Cox, H. R., 139
Craig, C. F., 88
Craigie, J., 140
Crawford, P. J., 143
Cromwell, Oliver, 23
Cullen, William, 31
Currie, William, 38
Cutter, John, 19

D

Dalldorf, G., 139
Davaine, C., 74
Davenport, C. B., 80
Davis, G. E., 139
Dawber, T. R., 134, 157
Dean, H. T., 157
Dempsey, E. W., 144
Dermer, Captain, 11
Devèze, Jean, 34, 36, 40

169

Dick, Everret, 61
Dick, George F., 140
Dick, Gladys H., 140
Diepgen, P., 28
Dingle, J. H., 138
Dochez, A. R., 91, 140
Douglass, William, 14
Downes, Jean, 146
von Drigalski, K. W., 90
Dublin, L. I., 80
Dubos, R. J., 118
Dyer, R. E., 139

E

Eddie, B., 145
Edwards, H. R., 134
Edwards, P. R., 141
Eldridge, W. W., 142
Eliot, Jared, 18
Emerson, Haven, 114, 152
Emmons, C. W., 142
Enders, J. F., 138
Evans, Alice C., 88, 141

F

Farr, William, 103
Feemster, R. F., 143
Ferrell, J. A., 147
Ferry, N. S., 88
Finke, L. L., 114, 130
Finlay, Carlos, 106
Flexner, Abraham, 83
Flexner, S., 88, 91, 115, 150
Flint, Austin, 93
Flournoy, T., 88
Fracastorius, 21, 39, 46, 48
Francis, E., 88
Francis, John, 55
Francis, Thomas, Jr., 138
Frankel, L. K., 80
Franklin, Benjamin, 18, 27
Fraser, F. R., 91
Freeman, A. W., 95, 100, 153
Frost, Wade Hampton, 75, 83, 85, 91, 92, 96, 100, 115, 126, 131, 147, 151
Furculow, M. L., 142

G

Galdston, I., 123
Galen, 18, 21
Galileo, 20
Garrison, F. H., 115
Gauld, R. L., 139
Gellis, S. S., 139
Ghon, A., 90
Gilliam, A. G., 139
Glover, J. W., 90
Godfrey, E. S., Jr., 131, 152

Goldberger, J., 102, 122
Goldmann, F., 146
Goodpasture, E. W., 143
Gookin, Daniel, 11
Gordon, J. E., 116, 122, 129, 134, 138, 146, 148, 157
Gordon, M. B., 18, 19
Gorgas, W. C., 82
Gover, Mary, 86
Graunt, J., 114, 130
Greenberg, M., 140
Griffits, T. H. D., 97
Griswold, Don M., 152

H

Habel, K., 138
Hackett, L. W., 145
Haeckel, E., 118
Hales, Stephen, 28
van Haller, Albrecht, 28, 32
Hamer, *Sir* William H., 103
Hamilton, Alice, 82
Hammon, W. M., 145
Hansen, A., 74
Hanson, 82
Hardy, A. V., 141
Harrison, R. G., 89
Havens, W. P., Jr., 138
Hayhurst, E. R., 82
Heidelberger, M., 140
Hektoen, Ludvig, 88
Henle, F. G. J., 74
Henle, W., 138
High, R. H., 142
Hill, H. W., 78, 93, 94, 95, 100, 115, 131, 147, 151
Hippocrates, 18, 21, 23, 41, 42, 49
Hirsch, August, 77, 118, 130
Hoffmann, F. L., 82
Howard, John, 32
Howard, W. T., 88
Howell, W. H., 84
Hudson, N. P., 138
Huebner, R. J., 140
Hunter, John, 28
Hutchinson, J., 11, 34

I

Ingalls, T. H., 157
Ipsen, J., 136

J

Janney, J. H., 134
Jennings, H. S., 120
Johnson, C. D., 143
Jordan, E. O., 122

K

Kastle, J. H., 91, 95
Kilborne, F. L., 79, 89, 97

Kilham, L., 138
King, W. W., 90
Kircher, Athenasius, 21, 46, 48, 114
Kittredge, G. L., 20
Knapp, R. E., 88
Knies, P. T., 146
Koch, Robert, 44, 74, 87, 90
Kober, George M., 82, 84
Koplik, H., 89
Krall, L. P., 134, 157
Kurland, L. T., 157

L

Lamb, B. H., 88
Lancefield, R. C., 140
Landsteiner, K., 88
Langmuir, A. D., 141
Lanoix, 58
La Roche, R., 29, 44, 45
Larson, C. L., 139
Lanza, A. J., 82
Lavinder, C. H., 100
Lazear, J. W., 88, 90
Leake, J. P., 100
Leavell, H. R., 146
Lee, F. S., 82
van Leeuwenhoek, Antony, 21, 46
Lenhart, C. H., 102
Le Prince, 97
Lettsom, J. C., 32
Levin, M., 157
Levy, E. C., 95
Lewis, P. A., 88
Lewis-Faning, E., 134
Light, R. U., 144
Lining, John, 29
Linnaeus, 46
Lloyd, W., 143
Loeffler, Friedrich, 90
Lombard, H. L., 133
Lotka, A. J., 103
Love, A. G., 80
Lovett, R. W., 92
Lumsden, L. L., 78, 91, 95

M

MacCallum, W. G., 90
Maclean, 38
MacLeod, C. A., 120, 138
Manson, P., 89
Marine, D., 101, 102
Martin, H. A., 58
Mason, Rev. J. M., 17
Massasoit, Indian Chief, 18
Mather, Cotton, 15, 17, 18, 20
Mather, Increase, 20
Maxcy, K. F., 100, 139
May, J. M., 144
McCoy, George, 88, 90, 131
McKay, F. S., 157

McMullen, J., 81
Mead, Richard, 22, 33, 39, 46, 49, 50
Meadors, G. F., 134, 157
Merrill, M., 136
Metz, C. W., 97
Meyer, K. F., 145
Milam, D. F., 134
Mitchell, John, 29
Mitchell, S. L., 41
Mitzmain, M. B., 97
Monroe, 31
Moore, F. E., 134, 157
Morgan, John, 31
Moriyama, I. M., 157
Moultrie, John, 27
Mountin, J., 159
Müller, P. T., 119
Munson, Elijah, 37
Munson, Eneas, 37
Murray, E. S., 139, 140
Murchison, Charles, 41

N

Neefe, J. R., 139
Negri, 58
Nichols, W. R., 101
Noguchi, H., 88
Norris, C., 88
Novy, F. G., 88
Nuttall, G. H. F., 88

O

Olson, B. J., 142
Oliphant, J. W., 139

P

Panum, P. L., 131
Pappenheimer, A. M., 88
Park, W. H., 90, 91, 131
Parsons, H. Franklin, 85
Pasteur, Louis, 74, 87, 114, 118
Paul, J. R., 143
Pearce, L., 143
Pearl, Raymond, 80
Pearson, Karl, 80
Penn, William, 24
Percy, George, 11
Perkins, J. E., 146
Perkins, R. G., 88
Perrott, G. St. J., 133
von Pettenkofer, Max, 41
Phair, J. J., 147
Philip, C. B., 151
Pike, G., 140
Plenciz, Marcus A., Sr., 46
Pollender, Aloys, 74
Pope, A. S., 126
Popper, E., 88

Price, 82
Puffer, Ruth R., 134

Q

Quinby, G. E., 141

R

Rauch, J. H., 56
Redi, Francesco, 114
Redman, John, 34
Reed, L. J., 134, 136
Reed, W., 86, 88, 90, 97
Rettger, L. F., 141
le Riche, H., 130
Richardson, M. W., 91
Rickard, E. R., 143
Ricketts, H. T., 88, 90
Riordan, J. R., 143
da Rosa, Ferreya, 29
Rose, Wickliffe, 84
Rogers, John, 26
Rosenau, Milton J., 81, 91, 95, 131, 151
Ross, John, 30
Ross, Ronald, 103
Rous, F. P., 89
Rumford, Count, 27, 50
Rush, Benjamin, 28, 31, 32, 33, 34, 35, 36, 38, 40, 42, 44, 47, 49, 50, 53, 54
Russell, P. F., 145

S

Saffron, M. H., 27
Sawyer, W. A., 139, 143, 145
Sayres, R. R., 82
Scamman, C. L., 119
Schereschewsky, J. W., 82
Schneider, F., Jr., 101
Schneider, H. A., 135, 144
Schoenbach, E. B., 147
Schrenk, H. H., 157
Schwentker, F. F., 134
Seaman, Valentine, 37
Sedgwick, W. T., 83, 93, 101
Shakespeare, O., 86
Shakespeare, William, 24
Shattuck, L., 11, 59, 60
Shaw, C. C., 151
Sherman, L., 140
Shippen, William, Jr., 32
Shryock, R. H., 19, 20, 27, 32
Sickles, G. M., 139
Simmons, J. S., 144, 150
Simpson, W. M., 145
Skaar, A. E., 143
Smadel, J. E., 151
Smillie, W. G., 138
Smith, C. E., 142
Smith, Elihu H., 37

Smith, H. E., 94
Smith, Stephen, 63, 71
Smith, Theobald, 79, 88, 89, 119, 136, 145
Snow, J., 114, 131, 159
Snyder, J. S., 139
Soper, F. L., 128, 143, 145
Soper, G. A., 91
Spence, J. C., 120
Stamps, P., 140
Stecker, M. L., 80
Sternberg, George M., 84, 90
Stevens, Dr., 55
Stiles, C. W., 88
Stokes, A., 138
Stokes, J., Jr., 139
Strode, G. K., 138
Strong, R. P., 88
Stuart-Anderson, B., 145
Sydenham, Thomas, 13, 21, 22, 23, 29, 44, 48, 49
Sydenstricker, E., 80, 86, 100, 102, 122, 133

T

Tandy, E. C., 24
Taylor, L. H., 93
Taylor, M. W., 94
Thoinot, L., 91
Thompson, Benjamin, 27
Thomson, G. W., 82
Tibbets, C., 133
Traub, R., 151
Tuck, D. H., 82
Turner, T. B., 134

V

Van Beneden, P. J., 118
Vaughan, Victor C., 83, 86
Vaughan, W. T., 122
Vesalius, 21
Villemin, J. A., 74
Von Ezdorf, R. H., 97

W

Warren, B. S., 80
Washington, George, 33, 37
Waterhouse, Benjamin, 58
Watt, J., 141
Wearn, J. F., 157
Weaver, G. H., 14
Webster, L. T., 135, 144
Webster, Noah, 12, 16, 29, 31, 34, 36, 37, 38, 39, 40, 41, 42, 43, 44, 47, 48, 49, 50, 54
Weinstein, L., 143
Welch, William H., 83, 84, 88
Wernstedt, W., 92
Wheeler, G. A., 102, 122

Wherry, W. B., 88, 90
Whipple, G. C., 79, 94
Wigglesworth, Edward, 67
Wilder, R. M., 139
Wilkerson, H. L. C., 134, 157
Williams, Huntington, 30
Wilson, D. B., 128
Wilson, L. B., 99
Winslow, C. E-A., 96, 125, 151
Winslow, Governor Edward, 18
Winthrop, General John, 25
Winthrop, Governor John, Jr., 18

Wolbach, S. B., 88
Worthington, John, 30
Wright, Carroll D., 80

Y

Yen, C. H., 140

Z

Zimmermann, Johann Georg, 32
Zingher, A., 91
Zinnser, Hans, 139
Zotta, G., 127

SUBJECT INDEX

A

Accidents, 76, 148, 157
Acclimatization, 106
Addiction to alcohol and drugs, 157
Administration, public health, 108, 152
Aedes calopus (Stegomyia), 99
Aedes egypti, 90
Africa, 128, 138, 143
Age of reason, 27
Agent, infectious, 77, 97, 115, 116
  nature of, 122
  of disease, 117, 118, 119, 120, 121, 122, 123, 124, 125, 127, 128, 134, 137-142, 144, 151, 155, 158, 160
Agriculture, 64, 136
  Department of, 79
Ague, 12, 61
  burning, 12
Aids, diagnostic, 75
Air, bad, 13
Alcohol, 32
  addiction to, 157
  as agent of disease, 116
America, 32, 52, 53, 72, 83, 94, 115, 128, 137, 139, 149, 151, 152, 156
American Academy of Arts and Sciences, 27
American Army, 122
American Association for the Advancement of Science, 139, 145, 146
American Epidemiological Society, 152
American Philosophical Society, 27
American Public Health Association, 90, 93, 125, 142, 146, 152
  Committee on Evaluation of Administrative Practice, 147
  Epidemiological Section, 152
American Red Cross, Medical Research Committee, 90
American Society of Tropical Medicine, 150
American Spelling Book, Webster, 36
Amherst, Massachusetts, 36
Anaphylaxis, 119

Anatomy, 28

Anatomy, 28
  pathologic, technic for field survey use, 143
Animal Industry, Bureau of, 79
Animalculae, of Plenciz, 46
Anomalies, congenital, 157, 160
Anopheles gambiae, 128
Anthrax, 74
Anthropology, social, 128
Antibiotics, 141, 142, 145
Anticontagionism, 46
Anticontagionists, 34
Antisepsis, 75
Appalachian Mountains, 62
Arch Street, decaying coffee on, 34, 36
Armed Forces Epidemiological Board, 148
Army Medical School, 84
  Service Graduate School, 151
Arsenic, 121, 125
Arthritis, rheumatoid, 134
Arthropods, transmission of infection by, 89, 90, 106, 119, 136
Asepsis, 75
Astrologers, 48
Athens, Greece, 127
Atlanta, Georgia, 153
Atmosphere, epidemic constitution of, 21, 22, 23, 33, 42, 44, 45, 48
Attack rates, secondary, 96, 126, 147
Aufklärung, 27
Australia, 139, 149
Autarcesis, 125, 143
Avignon, France, 22

B

Babesia (Piroplasma) begemina, 88
Bacilli, Brucella, 141
  colon, 91
  diphtheria, 90
  dysentery, 141
  tuberculosis, 82
  typhoid, 119, 140
  as disease agents, 116, 123
Bacillus, anthrax, 74
  colon, 91
  leprosy, 74

175

Bacillus—Cont'd
tubercle, 44, 125
typhoid, 107, 116, 122
Bacteria, 21, 46, 83, 140
Bacteriology, 69, 75, 83, 118, 119, 144
era of, 74
formal origin of, 118
Bacteriophages, 140
Baltimore, 30, 31, 37, 57, 64, 67, 134
Barbadoes Islands, 25, 29
Bartonella bacilliformis, 88
Batavia, New York, 100
Berkefeld filtrates, 89
Bible, 15
Bilious fevers, 12, 32, 35
Bills of Mortality, 43
Biochemistry, 151
Biology, 74, 75, 116, 119, 120
Biometry, 136
Biostatistics, 152
Birth rate, 62
Black Death, 25, 28
Black Sea Coast, 127
Blindness, 80
Blood-letting, 32
Board for the Investigation and Control of Influenza and Other Epidemic Diseases, U. S. Army, 148
Boards of health, 30, 31
Massachusetts State, Twenty-First Annual Report, 85
Michigan State, 79
Minnesota, 78
New York City, 60
Boophilus annulatus, tick, 89
Borrelia novyi, 88
Boston, 13, 14, 16, 17, 19, 20, 24, 25, 26, 27, 28, 30, 58, 64, 67, 81, 85, 96
scarlet fever in, 14, 15
smallpox inoculation in, 20
Botulism, 87
Brazil, 128
Brill's disease, 88, 89, 139
Bronchopneumonia in rodents, 88
Brucella, 141
abortus, 88
melitensis, 88
Brucellosis, 87, 145, 149
first outbreak attributable to goat's milk in the U. S., 87
Brunonian system in medicine, 28
ultra-position, 44
Buffalo, New York, 100

Burning fevers, 11
Bush Hill Hospital, 34, 40

C

Cadavers, dissection of, first law permitting, 20
Cairo, Egypt, 151
California, 57, 82, 87, 90, 153
Gold Rush, 57
Calorimeter, respiration, 75
Cambridge, England, 36
Camps, isolation, 25
Canada, 84, 152
Canadian border, 62
Cancer, 108, 123, 134, 135, 147, 154, 156, 157, 160
Carbon monoxide, presence in illuminating gas, 101
Caribbean area, 29
Caries, dental, 157
Carriers, 90, 91
animal, 41
cholera vibrio, 91
concept, 119
diphtheria, 91
human, 41, 47, 89, 106
inanimate, 41
insect, 39, 40, 41
meningococcus, 90
of poliomyelitis virus, 91
pneumococcus, 90, 91
typhoid, 86, 90, 91
well, 38
Case, clinical, 41, 89
secondary, 40
Cattle, Texas fever of, 79, 88, 89, 97
Causality of mass disease, 121, 122
in practice, 127, 128
multiple factors in, 125, 126
quantitative, 128
social factors in, 126
Causation, identification of multiple factors, 125
in practice, 127
multiple, of mass disease, 120, 121, 136, 141, 142, 143
Cemeteries, 56
Census, Bureau of, 79
federal, 80
population studies of, 79
reports of, 63, 64, 69, 70, 82
Century, Thirteenth, 25
Fourteenth, 25, 29, 48
Sixteenth, 25
Seventeenth, 12, 18, 19, 21, 24, 27, 29, 46, 114

Century—Cont'd
Eighteenth, 12, 19, 27, 29, 36, 40, 45, 49, 50, 52, 77
Nineteenth, 43, 46, 52, 56, 58, 59, 63, 72, 130, 131
Twentieth, 49, 59, 114, 145, 159
Characteristics, genetic, 135
immunological, 135
Charlatans, quacks and, 19
Charleston, South Carolina, 24, 27, 29
Charlestown, Massachusetts, 24
Chemistry, 74, 75
Chemoprophylaxis, of meningococcal infections, 147
Chemotherapy, 142, 145
Chester, Pennsylvania, 24
Child Hygiene, first Bureau of, 78
Children's Bureau, establishment of, 79
China, 85
Cholera, 47, 53, 55, 56, 57, 58, 59, 60, 61, 63, 69, 70, 79, 90, 124, 141, 144, 159
infantum and morbus, 70
vibrio, 91
Christophers Islands, 25
Cincinnati, Ohio, 100
Civil War, 59, 70
Climate and season, influence of, 22, 23
Clostridium welchii, 88
Coccidioidomycosis, 142
Coffee, decaying, on Arch Street, 34, 36
rotting, 53
Colic, Devonshire, 77
College of Medicine, Philadelphia, 31
College of Physicians, New Jersey, 28
Philadelphia, 28, 31, 34, 35, 36
Colonial Period, 15
Colonies, enlightenment comes to, 23
medical theory and medical practice in, prior to 1750, 18
physicians and practitioners in, 19
Colony, Connecticut, 26
Massachusetts, diphtheria in, 12
epidemic influenza in, 12
malignant fever in, 12
Columbia University, 28
Comets, 43
Commerce, Department of, 79
Commission on Respiratory Diseases, 138, 147

Committee on Evaluation of Administrative Practice, American Public Health Association, 147
Common cold, 126, 138, 155
Commonwealth Fund, 153
Communicability, experimental proof of, 74
laymen's concept of, 41
Communicable Disease Center, of the Public Health Service, 133
Complementarity, 136
Concept, epidemiological, 53, 55
Congenital anomalies, 157, 160
Conjunctivitis, ulcerative, 88
Connecticut, 15, 17, 18, 25, 26, 82, 94
diphtheria in, 1736, 15
pestilence in, 1712, 17
River, 12
scarlet fever in, 15
Consumption, 60, 70
miner's, 82
Contagion, 13, 21, 22, 23, 25, 27, 33, 34, 35, 38, 39, 40, 41, 43, 45, 46, 47, 48, 54
concept of, 21
control of, 25
specific, definition of, 38
vivum, 46
Contagionists, 22, 37, 40
Contagious sickness, 26
Contagium animatum, 46
Continent, North American, 29, 30
Convulsions, 70
Corynebacterium diphtheriae, 90
Cosmic forces, 54
Coughs, convulsive, of infants, 46
Countries, Scandinavian, 115
Croup, 70, 86
Coxsackie viruses, 139

D

Danube River, delta of, 127
Data, demographic, 130
morbidity, 80
D. D. T., 145
De Febre Flava, 27
Death rate, crude, in Chicago, 1845-1900, 59
in New Orleans, 1820-1900, 57
in New York City, 1810-1890, 55
in Philadelphia, 1810-1890, 53

Death rate—Cont'd
  infant, 69, 71
  rates, see Rates, death
Deaths by age groups, 67
  from throat distemper, 13
  from zymotic diseases, 1850 census, 69
  in 1850, 67
  seasonal distribution in the U. S., 61
Decomposition, miasmatic, 35
  organic, 22, 23, 42, 47
Deerfly fever, 88
Defect and disability, 155
Defects, physical, 81, 82, 83
  prevalence, 80, 81
Deficiency, nutritional, 123, 134, 155
Demography, 76, 79
Dengue fever, 88, 150
Denmark, 141
Dental caries, 157
  fluorosis, 157
Development, defective physical, 80
Devonshire colic, 77
Diabetes, 108, 123, 134, 147, 154, 155, 157
Diarrhea, 70, 94, 95, 141
  and enteritis, 53, 59
Dictionary-Webster, 36, 37
Diphtheria, 12, 14, 15, 29, 59, 61, 70, 79, 86, 91, 92, 96, 97, 100, 107, 108, 143
  antitoxin of, in well persons, 91, 143
  endemic, 96
  fatality rates in, 15
  in Connecticut, in 1736, 15
  in Massachusetts, 14, 15
  in New England, 12
  in New Jersey, in 1735, 15
  milk-borne, 87
  mortality rates, 86
Diplococcus pneumoniae, 90
Disability, 80, 81, 155
Discipline, biologic, 158
  scientific, 114, 117, 151
Disease, 106, 115, 130, 145
  communicable, 114, 116, 117, 118, 121, 134, 138, 148, 149, 155, 156, 159
  community, 115, 117, 126, 146, 158
  contagionistic theory of, 46
  contagious, 34, 56
  definition of, epidemiological, 117
  endemic, 133, 152

Disease—Cont'd
  epidemic, 46, 50, 57, 60, 64, 72, 152
  causation of, 42
  factors governing presence of, 23
  factors in production of, 116-120
  hookworm, 88, 150
  infectious, 59, 108, 119
  mass, 114, 115, 117, 118, 120, 121, 123, 125, 129, 130, 134, 135, 136, 142, 145, 146, 151, 153, 154, 155, 156, 157, 158, 159, 160
  causation, multiple of, 120, 121, 125, 126
  changing character of problems, 154-158
  experimental approach, 134, 135
  lines of approach to problems in Seventeenth Century, 114
  quantitative causality of, 128
  mental, 31
  muscardine, of silkworms, 74
  noncommunicable, organic, 156, 157
  prevention, 118, 119
  study of, 129
Diseases, arthropod-borne, 145, 155
  bacterial, 140
  chronic, 133, 136
  survey in Massachusetts, 133
  circulatory, 156
  communicable, 54, 55, 56, 96, 129, 134, 135, 136, 137, 145, 147, 148, 149, 154, 155, 156, 158, 159, 160
  contagious, 54
  deficiency, 75
  degenerative, 156
  diarrhoeal, of infancy, 53, 59, 60, 70
  epidemic, 53, 54, 60, 64
  preventive measures, practical, 23
  fungus, 74, 142
  infectious, 22, 56, 69, 74, 75, 76, 77, 80, 81, 83, 89, 106, 108, 119, 122, 137, 155, 159, 160
  control of, 23, 26, 56, 118, 119, 130
  dosage in, 107
  epidemiology of, 76
  mass phenomena of, 77, 106, 117, 154

Diseases, infectious—Cont'd
  prevention of, 56, 60
  transmission, 69
  metabolic, 156
  miasmatic, 54
  non-infectious, 76, 77, 101, 102,
    107, 134, 160
  occupational, 82
  of old age, 156
  of skin, 21
  pestilential, 54, 58, 67
  protozoal, 141
  respiratory, 60, 85, 138
  rickettsial, 139, 140, 148
  social, 157
  virulent, 54
  virus, 137, 138, 139
  of man and animals, 89
  zymotic, 53, 54, 56, 60, 67, 69,
    70

Disinfection, 89

Disorders, emotional and mental,
  135, 160
  endocrine, 75, 123, 144
  mental, 123, 148, 153, 157, 160
  neuropsychiatric, 155

Distemper, Eastern, 13
  throat, 13, 14, 16

District of Columbia, 78, 79, 84, 95

Dosage, community, 142

Drug addiction, 157

Durham, Connecticut, 14

Dysentery, 12, 29, 38, 42, 44, 45,
  46, 55, 59, 70, 94, 95, 141,
  150
  epidemics of, 29, 95
  water-borne, 95

E

Eastern distemper, 13

Eastern Health District, Baltimore,
  134

Eberthella typhosa, 90

Ecology, 116, 117, 118, 119, 145,
  158
  definition of, 116
  formal origin of, 118
  medical, 116-120

Edinburgh, 27, 28, 31

Education, medical, 83
  professional, 83
  public health, 147

Elephantiasis, 46

Employment of the Free Male
  Population, 1850 Census,
  64

Encephalidites, arthropod-b o r n e,
  141, 145

Encephalitis lethargica (nona), 87,
  115

England, 19, 20, 23, 24, 36, 82, 85,
  94, 95, 103
  Edward III of, 24
  medical training of colonials in,
    19
  smallpox, inoculation against, 20

English Friendly Societies, 80

English Plague Commission, 90

Englishmen, 11

Enlightenment comes to the colonies, 27

Enteritis, 53, 59, 70

Entomology, Division of, 79

Environment, 21, 22, 23, 54, 69, 97,
  116, 117, 118, 122, 123,
  126, 128, 132, 137, 154,
  158, 159
  as factor in disease, 117, 123, 124,
    125, 127, 135, 137, 143,
    144-146, 158, 159
  biologic, 116, 124, 128, 144
  epidemiologic influence of, 124,
    144, 145, 146
  categories of, 124, 144
  physical, 114, 116, 119, 124, 127,
    135, 144
  relationship to host and parasite,
    116-120
  social component, 116, 124, 125,
    127, 135, 144, 146, 159

Epidemic constitution, 118
  of atmosphere, 21, 22, 23, 29,
    33, 42, 43, 44, 45, 48, 49,
    50

Epidemics, 11, 13, 15, 29, 37, 40,
  42, 43, 45, 47, 48, 52, 54,
  56, 58, 62, 69, 72, 76, 77,
  84, 86, 87, 92, 93, 94, 95,
  98, 100, 102, 103, 107,
  114, 121, 127, 128, 130,
  131, 133, 135, 141
  application of statistical methods
    to, 103
  causes of, 56, 62, 69
  devastating, 12
  milk-borne, 86, 87, 94
  of cruell diseases, 11
  period of great, 52
  theory of, 102, 115
  water-borne, 86, 93, 94, 95

Epidemiologic method, 129-136

Epidemiological Society, of London,
  136, 151

Epidemiologist, 78, 79, 102, 106, 107, 108, 119, 126, 141, 145, 147, 148, 149, 150, 151, 159
  first with state board of health, 78
  with Public Health Service, 153
Epidemiologists, 47
  American, 106, 108, 149, 150
Epidemiology, a scientific discipline, 151
  advances in, 106
  American, 105, 114, 137-146, 152, 159
  evolution of, 92, 107
  an analytical discipline, 131
  as profession, 151-154
  as medical ecology, 116
  as science, 76
  comparative, 136
  concepts and basis for, 114-120
  current and modern, 76-78
  definition of, 117
  evolution of American, 92
  experimental, 129, 134, 135, 160
    definition of, 135
  first chair of, 151
    department of, 83
    division of, 78
  field investigations, 92
    study, historical-geographical concept of, 130
  future in, 159
  growth of, 78, 108
  ideal methodology of, 76
  important principles established, 89
  in America, 11
  international interests, 148-149
  medical approaches to, 18-23
  methods of study, 130-136
    clinical contribution, 132
    collection of demographic data, 130
    comparative method, 130
    field review, 134
    field study, pattern for, 132
    field survey, 133
    historical development, 130-135
    laboratory participation, 132
    team effort, 133
  military, 148, 160
  modern concepts, 76
  of health, 136
  operational, 133, 146, 150, 152, 160
  operational activities, 146-151, 152

Epidemiology—Cont'd
  scientific, 44
  scope of, 76
  Section, American Public Health Association, 152
  serological, 143
  state of, in 1800, 45
  trends in methodology, 136-137
  tropical, 149, 150, 151
  unit of, 76, 126
  Webster's interest in, 37
  X factor in, 49, 50
Era, bacteriological, 45, 74, 75, 76, 79, 108, 109, 114
  advances in human affairs, 76
  colonial, 11
  statistical, 79
Eruptions, volcanic, 43, 54
Erysipelas, 58, 60, 70, 140
  from vaccination transmission, 58
Eskimos, 143
Etiology, 118, 120, 121
  American contributions to, 77, 87, 88, 89
  definition of, 120
  in disease of the individual, 120
  types of, 120
Europe, 19, 25, 27, 28, 32, 33, 63, 83, 85, 92, 94, 137, 155
  medical training of colonials in, 19
  northern, 25
Examination, medical, of school children, 81
Exeter, New Hampshire, 13
Exhalations, earth, 22
  marsh, 34
  pestilential, 36
  putrid, vegetable and animal, 35
Expectation of life, in U. S., 67, 68

F

Factors affecting disease occurrence, environmental, 54, 69, 71
  epidemiological, 56
  nutritional, 62
  primary, as governing presence of epidemic disease, 23
  social, 62, 63
Fallacies, epidemiological, 56
Famine, 11
Fatality rates, scarlet fever, in Boston, 14, 15
Fermentation, 53
Fever, De Febre Flava, 27
  deerfly, 88
  dengue, 88
  intercurrent, 21
  intermittent, 70

Fever—Cont'd
  intestinal, 70
  malignant, 12, 26, 44
  Oroya, 88
  Pepperill, 29
  pestilential, 21, 26
  Q, 139
  remittent, 44, 70
  rheumatic, 46
  three day, 85
  typhus, 29, 38, 41, 45, 71, 88, 89,
    139, 146
Fevers, bilious, 12, 35, 42
  and remitting, 32
  burning, 11
  intercurrent, 21
  intermittent, 41, 44, 46, 55
  malignant, 46
  pestilential, 46, 48
  petechial, 46
  remittent, 41, 44
Filaria bancrofti, 89
Filth, 24, 60, 62, 114
Filtrates, Berkefeld, 89
Fleas, 39, 90, 146
Flies, 62, 69, 86
Florida, 99
Fluorosis, dental, 157
Fluxes, 11
Fomites, 22, 38, 40
  disinfection of, 22
Foot, deformity of, 80
Forces, cosmic, 54
Fractures, 123
Framingham, Massachusetts, 81, 134
France, 23, 29, 58, 81, 115
Fungus, 74

G

Galvanometer, string, 75
Galveston, Texas, 84
Gas gangrene, 88
  poisoning, 101, 108
Genetics, human, 128
Geneva, Switzerland, 149
Geography, 76
  medical, 114
Georgetown Medical School, 84
Geriatrics, 156
Germ, 41, 45, 49, 115
  theory, 21, 74
German measles, 160
Germany, 82, 83, 103, 115
Germs, of Plenciz, 1762, 46
God, wrath of, 15, 16, 33
Goiter, 81
  endemic, experimental studies,
    101, 102, 108

Göttingen, 28
Gout, 46
Great Britain, 83, 115, 122, 141
Greece, 127
Greenland, 85
Groton, Connecticut, 26
Gulf of Mexico, 62

H

Hagerstown, Maryland, 133
Halifax, Nova Scotia, 57
Halteridium, a bird parasite, 90
Hanover, Germany, 32
Hartford, Connecticut, 36
Harvard University, 28, 151
Havana, Cuba, 99
Haverhill, Massachusetts, 16
  diphtheria in, 14
  throat distemper in, 13
Hawaii, 150
Health, boards of, 30, 31, 45, 60,
    78
  lay, 56
  Massachusetts State, Twenty-
    First Annual Report, 85
  Michigan State, 79
  Minnesota, 78
  New York City, 60
  commissioner of Boston, 81
  commissioners of, 30, 60
  Committee of, in Baltimore, 30,
    31
  in New York, 30
  in Philadelphia, 30
  department, 30, 31, 78, 94, 133,
    147, 151, 152, 153
  city, 78
  county, 78
  first organized, 30
  officer, 31, 60, 78, 83, 92, 147
  organizations, voluntary, 153,
    154
  public, 31, 47, 60, 78, 79, 83,
    101, 102, 105, 119, 130,
    146, 147, 148, 151, 152,
    156
  units, county, 78
  wardens, 61
Hearing, defective, 83
Heart, defects of, 80
  disease, 80, 154, 155, 156, 157
  study, Framingham, 134
Hemophilus bronchisepticus, 88
Hepatitis, infectious, 138
  serum, 139
Herd, immunological characteristics
    of, 135
  reactions, 151

Hernia, 80
Hibbing, Minnesota, 95
Histoplasmosis, 142
Hookworm disease, 78, 88, 150
Hospital, Pennsylvania, 28, 31
Hospitals, isolation, 25
Host, 96, 108, 116, 117, 118, 119,
    120, 122, 124, 125, 126,
    127, 128, 132, 135, 137,
    142, 143, 144, 158
  factor, in causation of disease,
    123, 125, 142, 143
Host-parasite-environment relation-
    ships, 116-120
Housing, 60, 62, 63, 69, 71, 125,
    146
Howard Association, 84
Hygiene, Child, first Bureau of, 78
  first Special Laboratory, 83
  industrial, 79, 82
Hygienic Laboratory, of Public
    Health Service, 131, 153

I

Illinois, 82
Illness, 81
  surveys, 80
Immigration from Europe, 63
Immunity, 92, 107, 125
  acquired, 38, 40
  and aggregation of population, 91
  antitoxin in diphtheria, 91, 107
  definition of, 125
  from subclinical infection, 91, 106
  specific, 123, 125, 144
  theory of, 106, 107
Immunization, active, 141
  latent, 142
Immunology, 119
Incubation period, extrinsic, 97
Index case, 126
Indian Plague Commission, 149
Indians, 11, 12, 52
Industrial hygiene, 79, 82
Industry, 64
Infection, 25, 37, 39, 40, 41, 42, 43,
    48, 69, 89, 91, 98, 106,
    114, 120, 122, 123, 125,
    131, 135, 142, 149
  chemical, 40
  chronic, 134
  importation of, 37, 39
  latent, 132, 142
  reservoirs of, 139
    in animals, 77
  resistance to, definition, 125
  salmonella, 149

Infection—Cont'd
  sources of, 119
  subclinical, 91, 96
    immunity from, 91, 106
  theory of Webster and contem-
    poraries, 41
Infections, 25, 70
  arthropod-borne, 145
  concealed, 77
  intestinal, 70, 141, 154
  of infancy, 70
  meningococcal, 147
  pestillential, 25
  pyogenic, 140
  salmonella, 149
  venereal, 21, 46, 147, 155
Influenza, 12, 21, 23, 29, 37, 40,
    44, 48, 49, 75, 84, 85, 86,
    100, 108, 115, 122, 138,
    141, 149
  attack rates, 86
  death rates, 86
  epidemic, in New England, 1697-
    1698, 12
  of, 1789 and 1790, 37
  pandemic of, 1918-1919, 85, 86
Injections, parenteral, of antigens,
    143
Injuries, 125, 157, 158
  accidental, 147
  mass, 122, 123, 155, 158, 160
  military, 157
  traumatic, 121, 148
Insanitation, 47
Institute of Technology, Massa-
    chusetts, 83
Institutes of Health, National, U. S.
    Public Health Service, 78,
    153
Institutes of Medicine, Philadelphia,
    31
Insusceptibility, inherent, 125, 143
Intercurrent fevers, 21
Interior, Department of, 79
Intermittent fevers, 44, 46, 55, 70
International Health Division,
    Rockefeller Foundation,
    138, 150
Intestinal fever, 70
Iodine therapy in goiter, 102
Iowa, 87, 100
Isolation, 21, 22, 27, 45, 55, 56, 89
  hospitals, 25
  of microorganisms, 75
  procedures, 21
Italy, 42

J

Jamestown, Virginia, 11
Jaundice, homologous serum, 139
Johns Hopkins School of Hygiene
and Public Health, 83, 151
Johns Hopkins University, 83

K

Kellogg, W. K., Foundation, 154
Kentucky, 81
Key West, Florida, 99
Kingston, New Hampshire, throat
distemper in, 1735, 13

L

Labor, Department of, 79, 80
Laboratory, Hygienic, at University
of Pennsylvania, 83
public health, 78, 147
first, 78
Law, Mendel's, 75
Lawrence, Massachusetts, 93
Lead as agent of disease, 116, 123
League of Nations, Health Section,
149
Legislation relating to health mat-
ters, 23, 24, 25, 26, 30
Leishmaniasis, 143
Leprosaria, 25
Leprosy, 21, 25, 46, 74, 76
pandemic of, 25
Leptospirosis, 145
Lerida, 22
Leyden, 28
Lice, body, 90
Life, community, 63
expectation of, in the U. S., 68
table technic, 126
Liver, viscerotome specimens of, 143
London, 29, 32, 33, 136, 149, 151
London Epidemiological Society,
151
London, John Hunter's Anatomy
Museum, 28
Lowell, Massachusetts, 93

M

Macedonia, 127
Maine, diphtheria in, 14
throat distemper in, 13, 15
Malaria, 12, 32, 35, 42, 45, 47, 55,
59, 62, 71, 89, 97, 127,
128, 141, 145, 147, 150,
151
Malaya, 151
Malignant fever, 12, 46
Mankato, Minnesota, 93, 94, 95
Marseilles, 25, 39

Marseilles—Cont'd
quarantine regulations in, 1373,
25
Maryland, 30, 100
laws of, for 1893, 30
Mason City, Iowa, 100
Mass disease, changing character of
problems, 154-160
diseases, of childhood, 156
experimental approach, 135
phenomenon of disease, 76, 106,
114, 131, 151
of health, 76
Massachusetts, 11, 12, 14, 15, 24,
25, 30, 79, 80, 81, 83, 87,
92, 93, 101, 131, 133
Bay, 52
first law permitting dissection of
cadavers, 20
Institute of Technology, 83
scarlet fever in, 15
State Board of Health, Twenty-
First Annual Report, 85
state gas commission, 101
throat distemper in, 13
tribe of Indians, 11
Measles, 21, 23, 29, 35, 38, 44, 45,
46, 47, 48, 54, 70, 88, 89,
101, 103, 108, 158
German, 160
Medical care, 146
in colonies, 18
Medical Repository, a journal, 28
Medical school at Edinburgh, 27
Medical schools, American, 83, 151
colonial, 28
Medicine, application of the experi-
mental method, 20
Brunonian system, 28
Institutes of, Philadelphia, 31
men, 19
practitioners of, in colonial times,
18
preventive, 146, 148, 151, 158,
159
tropical, 149, 150, 151
Memphis, Tennessee, 84
Mendel's law, 75
Meningitis, cerebrospinal, 60, 70,
87, 115
Meningococci, 140
Menstruation, 143
Mental disorder, epidemiology of,
148
Mephitic vapors, 43
Merrimack River, 13, 93

Meteorology, 76
Meteors, 54
Method, epidemiologic, 129-136, 158
  epidemiological, 130
  microbiologic, in mass disease, 114, 115
Methods, epidemiological, 77, 137
  applied to noninfectious diseases, 101, 108
Metropolitan Life Insurance Company, 80, 81
Mexican typhus, 88
Miasma, 53
Miasmata, 53, 54, 70
Miasmatists, 37
Miasms, 33, 34, 42, 43, 44, 45, 47, 49
Michigan, 82
  University of, 83
Microbes of van Leeuwenhoek, 46
Microbiological Congress, Third International, 119
Microbiologists, American, 137, 138
Microbiology, 87, 88, 89, 103, 131, 142
Microfilaria, 89
Microorganisms, 75, 88, 89, 92, 103, 107, 114, 122, 125, 139
  proof of specific relationship of, to disease, 88, 89
Middle Ages, 27
Migration, 64
Milbank Memorial Fund, 146, 153, 157
Milk, 41, 86, 87, 94, 95, 96
  -borne epidemics, 86, 87, 94
  standards, 92
Mines, Bureau of, 79, 82
Ministers, of gospel, 14, 17, 33
Minnesota, 78, 87, 93, 95, 131, 147
  University Agricultural College, 95
Mississippi River, 58
Missouri, 82
Mithriditization, 91
Mobile, Alabama, 98
Montana, 153
Montgomery County, New York, 37
Morbidity data, 80, 152
Mortality, Bills of, 43
  data, 152
  infant, studies on, 79
  rate, infant, 63, 69
Mosquitoes, 33, 71, 89, 97, 98, 103, 104, 105

Mosquitoes—Cont'd
  Culex, 89
  in yellow fever, 34, 97, 98, 99
Motivations, social, 146
Mount Vernon, Virginia, 33
Multiple sclerosis, 154, 157
Mumps, 138, 139
  in monkeys, 143
Mycobacterium tuberculosis, 88

N

Narragansett, smallpox in, 12
Natal, South Africa, 128
National Foundation for Infantile Paralysis, 139, 154
National Institutes of Health, U. S. Public Health Service, 78, 153
National Tuberculosis Association, 81, 82
Nativity of population (four largest cities) in U. S., 1850 census, 64
Navy, U. S., 85
  Epidemiological Unit, 150
Necator americanus, 88
Negroes, 63, 64, 81
Neisseria meningitidis, 90
Neoplasms, 155
New England, 11, 12, 16, 52, 134
  epidemic of influenza in, 1697-1698, 12
New Hampshire, 14, 45
  diphtheria in, 14
  throat distemper in, 13
New Haven, 30, 36, 37, 39, 40
New Jersey, 15, 79
  college of physicians of, 28
  diphtheria in, 1735, 15
  State Medical Society, 28
New London, 26
New Netherlands, 25
New Orleans, 57, 58, 84, 98
New York, 12, 17, 19, 25, 28, 29, 30, 36, 37, 38, 40, 55, 57, 60, 64, 67, 78, 80, 85, 86, 87, 89, 90, 91, 107, 131, 138, 140
  yellow fever in, 1668, 12
New York Academy of Medicine, 146
New York Quarantine Station, 91
  Sanitary Association, 1857, 60
New York, state of, 30, 82, 87, 93, 100, 131
Noncontagious, 14
Norfolk, Virginia, 30, 37

North America, 34, 155
North Boston, New York, 93
Nose and throat affections, 83
Nutrition, 69, 144, 151, 153, 156

O

Occupations, deaths by, 82
Office International d'Hygiene, 149
Oiling of floors and bedding, 147
Oklahoma, 78
Ophthalmia, 21
Oroya fever, 88
Orwood, Mississippi, 97

P

Pacific Ocean, 62
Panama Canal Zone, 150
Panama, Isthmus of, 106
Pan American Sanitary Bureau, 149
Pandemic, 25, 49, 84, 86, 100, 115,
    122
Paralysis in poliomyelitis, 143
Parasite, 97, 105, 116, 118, 119,
    120, 124, 142
  in yellow fever, 104, 105
  relationship to host and environ-
    ment, 116-120
Parasitism, 119, 120, 145
Paratyphoid fever, 86
Paris, 22, 48, 49
Pasteurella tularensis, 88
Pathology, experimental, definition
    of, 134, 135
  historical and geographical, 77,
    108, 114, 144
  mass, 134, 137
  social, 108
Peaks, epidemic, 56
Pellagra, 102, 108, 123
  field studies, 102, 108
Pennsylvania Hospital, 28, 31
Pennsylvania, University of, 28, 83
Penrith, England, 94
Pepperill fever, 29
Pestilence, 15, 22, 38, 39, 43, 71
  in Connecticut, in 1712, 17
  that walketh in darkness, 11
Pestilential fever, 21, 26, 46, 48
Petechial fever, 46
Pharmacology, 136
Philadelphia, 17, 24, 27, 28, 29, 30,
    31, 33, 34, 37, 38, 40, 47,
    48, 52, 53, 55, 57, 64, 67,
    93
  College of Medicine, 31
  of Physicians, 28, 31, 34, 35, 36
Philippines, 150
Phthisis, 21, 46

Physician, 13, 14, 18, 19, 20, 21, 23,
    28, 31, 33, 34, 37, 38, 41, 45,
    49, 54, 55, 61, 62, 75, 83,
    84, 137, 157
Physics, 74, 75
Physiology, 28, 151
Pilgrims, 11, 52
  at Plymouth, 11
von Pirquet test, 75
Piscataqua River, 12
Plague, 11, 21, 25, 26, 28, 29, 33,
    36, 38, 39, 40, 41, 42, 45,
    47, 48, 49, 55, 87, 90, 124,
    140, 145, 146
  Laboratory, U. S. Public Health
    Service, 152
  tractates, 49
  tracts, 21, 48
Plagues, 17, 42, 43, 52
Pleurisy, 54
  putrid, 16
Plymouth, Massachusetts, 18
  landing, 11
  Pilgrims at, 11
Plymouth, Pennsylvania, 93
Pneumococci, 88, 140
Pneumonia, 53, 59, 61, 62, 70, 85,
    90, 100, 106, 147, 155,
    156
  and influenza, as a cause of death,
    155
  primary atypical, 138
Poisoning, 100, 121, 160
  by illuminating gas, 101, 108
  deaths from, 101
Poisons, industrial, 135
Poliomyelitis, 87, 88, 91, 92, 100,
    108, 115, 126, 139, 143,
    144
  cases and deaths, 87
  transmission of, 100
  virus of, 126
    in healthy persons, 91, 92
Pollution, atmospheric, 157
Population, 160
  character and migration, 119
  comparison of increase of urban
    and rural, 1820-1940, 67
  employment of free male, over 15
    years of age, 1850 census,
    64
  in 1850, 63, 64
  in U. S., age distribution, 1850
    compared with 1940, 64,
    65

Population—Cont'd
  mass disease and, 121
  migration, 64
  nativity, 1850, 64
  pressures, 146, 153
  rate of growth, 1780-1948, 66, 67
  surveys, 100
Porto Rico, 150
Posture, faulty, 83
Practice, epidemiological, 137, 138, 153
  medical, in colonies, 18, 19
  quacks and charlatans, 19
Practitioners of medicine, 18, 19
Preacher, 16, 33
Pregnancy, 143
Preventive medicine, 146, 148, 151, 158, 159
  first department in medical school, 151
  military, 148
Preventive Medicine Service, Office of Surgeon General, 148
Primary atypical pneumonia, 138
Protozoa, 46
Providence, Rhode Island, 40, 108, 126
Provinces, Eastern, 14
Public health, 31, 47, 60, 78, 79, 83, 101, 102, 105, 119, 130, 146, 147, 148, 151, 152, 154, 156, 158, 159, 160
  education, 147
  laboratory, first, 78
  nurse, 133
  officers, 31, 60, 78, 83, 92, 147
  schools of, 151
Public Health Organization, progress during Bacteriological Era, 78
Public Health Reports, 85, 94, 97
Public Health Service, 78, 79, 80, 81, 82, 95, 97, 100, 131, 133, 152, 153
  Communicable Disease Center, Atlanta, 133, 153
  Hygienic Laboratory, 131, 153
  Institutes of Health, 78, 153
  Plague Laboratory, California, 153
  Rocky Mountain Spotted Fever Laboratory, Montana, 153

Puerperal sepsis, 140
Puerto Rico, 150
Putrefaction, 34, 41, 42

Q

Q fever, 139
Quacks and charlatans, 19
Quarantine, 14, 23, 26, 27, 35, 36, 45, 47, 55, 61, 97
  in Colonial Era, 23
  maritime, 25, 55
  measures, 35, 97
  physicians in Baltimore, 30, 31
  regulations, 25
    Marseilles, 1373, 25
    Ragusa, 1377, 25
    Venice, 1374, 25
  station, Marseilles, 25
Quarantine Act of London of 1825, 55
Quarantine and Sanitary Convention of 1857, 55
Quarantine Station, New York, 91
Quinine, 71

R

Rabies, 29, 46, 145
Ragusa, quarantine regulations, in 1377, 25
Rate, attack, secondary, 96, 97, 126, 147
  birth, 62
  death, 60, 62, 63, 71, 72
  fatality, 142
  morbidity, 72, 142
  mortality, 142
    infant, 63, 69, 79
Rates, incidence, 76
Rats, 39, 90, 139, 146
Reactions, herd, 151
Reason, Age of, 27
Reformers, 32
Reforms, sanitary, 63, 70
Registration area for deaths, 79, 82, 85, 86, 87
  of births, 79
  of deaths, 79
Regulations, boards of health, lay, 56
  sanitary, 24
Relapsing fever, American, 88
Remittent fever, 44, 70
Reporting of diseases, 79
Research, microbiological, 137
Reservoirs, animal, 106, 124, 155
  of infection, 139, 142, 155
  plant, 124

Respiratory disease, 60, 147
  mortality from, 85
  outbreak of, in 1655, 12
Revolution, industrial, 62
Revolutionary War, 17, 32
Rheumatic fever, 46
Rhode Island, 12, 19, 119, 126
  burning ague in, in 1723, 12
Rialta, Italy, 58
Rickettsial diseases, 139, 148
Rickettsialpox, 140
Rickettsia rickettsii, 88
Richmond, Virginia, 95
Rockefeller Foundation, 78, 83, 153
  International Health Division, 138, 150
  Sanitary Commission, 78
Rocky Mountain spotted fever, 88, 90, 99, 106, 108, 139
  Laboratory, Montana, 153
Romania, 127, 134
Rutland, Vermont, 87

S

Salem, Massachusetts, 24
Salmonella infection, 149
San Francisco, California, 87
Sanitary Commission of 1849, 59
Sanitary Conference of Paris, in 1851, 54
Sanitary Conventions, 1857-1860, 70
Sanitary engineering, 152
Sanitary Police, first established by King John II, of France, 23
Sanitary science, 83
  survey, engineering, 95
  of New York City, 71
Sanitation, 22, 23, 24, 26, 27, 36, 47, 55, 62, 71
  community, 71
  control of disease by, 24
  environmental, 55, 144
  in American colonies, 24
  in Colonial Era, 23
  in England, in 1297, 23
Saugus, Massachusetts, smallpox in, 12
Scabies, 21, 46
Scarlet fever, 14, 15, 29, 37, 46, 52, 54, 59, 70, 79, 86, 92, 96, 97, 100, 101, 108, 134, 140, 143
  endemic, 96
  epidemic, in 1793, 37
  fatality rates in Boston, 14, 15
  in Connecticut, 15
  in Massachusetts, 15

Scarlet fever—Cont'd
  milk-borne, 87
  mortality rates, 87
Schick test, 75, 91, 107
Schistosomiasis, 150
School of Hygiene and Public Health, Johns Hopkins University, 83
Schools, medical, 28
  Philadelphia, 1765, 28
  New York, 1768, 28
  Boston, 1783, 28
Science, 74, 120
  medical, 56
  modern experimental, 27
Sciences, basic, 75, 76, 146
  biological, 128, 132, 133, 136
  medical, 76, 132
  physical, 120
  sanitary, 83, 128
  social, 126, 128, 133, 136
Sclerosis, multiple, 154, 157
Scotland, 28
Scrub typhus, 139, 151
Season, influence of, 33, 35
Secondary attack rate, 96, 97, 126, 147
  history of, 96, 126
Septic acid, 41, 43
  sore throat, 52, 95, 96
  epidemics of, 95, 96
  milk-borne outbreak of, 95, 96
Sermon of Cotton Mather, 15
Sewage or wastes, 23, 24, 62, 69
Sheffield, Massachusetts, 37
Shellfish, 86, 92, 95
Shigella, group, 88
Siberia, 84
Silkworms, muscardine disease of, 74
Sin, 15, 16, 17
Slavery, 32
Slaves, 63
Smallpox, 11, 12, 20, 21, 23, 25, 26, 29, 35, 38, 41, 44, 45, 46, 47, 52, 53, 54, 55, 56, 57, 58, 59, 60, 61, 70, 79, 87
  epidemic in New England, 1677-1678, 12
  in 1721, 20
  epidemics of, in Boston, 1702, 1721, 12
  fatality rates, 87
  in Europe between 1665 and 1675, 12
  inoculation against, 20
  mortality rates, 87

Society, American Philosophical, 27
Society of Physicians Anti Inoculator, 20
Sociology, 76
Sore throat, streptococcal, 140
South America, 143
South Carolina, 24, 102
    special orders regarding sanitation, 24
Spanish American War, 83, 86, 150
Spontaneous generation, doctrine of, 74
St. Peter, Minnesota, 95
Stamford, Connecticut, 94
Standards, bacteriological, for water, milk and shellfish, 92
State Gas Commission of Massachusetts, 101
Statistics, 76
    an approach to problem of mass disease, 114
    vital, 79
Stegomyia (Aedes), 103, 104, 105
Stimulus, 54
Stratford-on-Avon, Court Rolls of, 1552, 24
Streptococcal sore throat, 140
Streptococci, hemolytic, group A, 140
Streptococcus in septic sore throat, 95
Streptococcus mucosus, 88
Studies, Hagerstown, 133
Sub-infection, 91
Subclinical infection, 91
Sulfonamides, 141
Surgeon General, U. S. Army, 84, 148
Surgery, 75
Survey, illness, 80
    National Health, 133
Survival of host, 118
    of parasite, 118, 120
Sweden, 92
Swellings, 11
Syphilis, 54, 58, 76, 134, 143
    vaccination transmission, 58
System, Brunonian, 28

T

Tabardillo, 88
Tampa, Florida, 99
Teeth, defective, 83
Teething, 70
Tennessee, 84, 134
Tertian fever, 44
Test, mouse protection, in yellow fever, 143

Test—Cont'd
    neutralization, in poliomyelitis, 143
    von Pirquet, 75
    Schick, 75, 91, 107
    skin, for mumps, 143
    tuberculin, 143
    Wassermann, 75
    Widal, 75, 89
Tests, immunological, 143
Texas, 87
    fever, of cattle, 79, 88, 89, 97
Theology, 18
Theory, epidemiological, 17, 75, 76, 77, 102, 131, 137
    germ, 21, 74
Therapy, antibiotic, 141, 142
    chemotherapeutic, 142
    sulfonamide, 141
Three day fever, 85
Throat distemper, 13, 14, 15, 16
    in Haverhill, Massachusetts, 13, 16
        analysis, statistical, of, 16
    in Kingston, New Hampshire, 13
    in Maine, 13, 15
    in Massachusetts, 13
    in New Hampshire, 13, 15
Thyroid gland, 102
Tick, Boöphilus annulatus, 89
    wood, Dermacentor andersoni, 90
Ticks, 89, 90, 97, 99, 100
Tobacco, 32
Tonsillectomy, 143
Tools, diagnostic, 75
Toxin, diphtheria, 143
Trachoma, 81
Traite de la peste, 39
Transmission of infection, 142
    by arthropods, 89, 90, 106, 119, 136
    by healthy carriers, 89, 90, 91, 106
    by patients, 69
    modes of, 89, 119, 134, 135, 145
    person to person, 54, 56, 107
    transovarian, 90
Transylvania highlands, 127
Trauma, 157, 160
Trench fever, 90
    foot, 157
Triatoma megista, 90
Trypanosomiasis, South American, 90
Tuberculin test, 143

Tuberculosis, 21, 44, 53, 59, 60, 70, 74, 76, 81, 82, 103, 106, 119, 125, 126, 134, 146, 147, 153, 154, 155, 156
    death rates, 60
Tularemia, 145
Tumor of fowls, 89
Typhoid fever, 12, 42, 45, 53, 54, 59, 61, 62, 63, 70, 78, 84, 86, 89, 91, 92, 93, 94, 95, 106, 107, 108, 141, 151
    cases and deaths, 86, 93, 94
    endemic, 94, 95, 107
    epidemics of, 93, 94, 95
    from eating raw oysters, 94
    milk-borne, 86, 94
    transmission, 93, 94, 95
    water-borne, 86, 93, 94, 95
Typhoid Mary, 91
Typhus fever, 29, 38, 41, 45, 60, 71, 89, 139, 146
    Brill's disease, 88, 89, 139
    classical, 139
    malignant, 29
    Mexican, 88
    murine, 139
    recurrent louse-borne, 139
    scrub, 139, 151

U

United Nations Relief and Rehabilitation Association, 149
United States Army, disability records of, 80
    Medical School, 84
    Medical Service Graduate School, 151
    prevalence of tuberculosis in, 82
    Typhus Commission, 140, 148
    Yellow Fever Commission, 106
United States Marine Hospital Service, 45
United States Navy, 85
    Epidemiological Unit, 150
United States Public Health Service, 78, 79, 80, 81, 82, 86, 95, 97, 100, 131, 133, 152
    Communicable Disease Center, Atlanta, 133, 153
    Hygienic Laboratory, 131, 153
    Institutes of Health, 78, 153
    Plague Laboratory, California, 153
    Rocky Mountain Spotted Fever Laboratory, Montana, 153

Universe, epidemiologic, 150, 159
University of Michigan, 83
University of Minnesota Agricultural College, 95
University of Pennsylvania, 28, 83
Urbanization, 63, 67
Utah, 88

V

Vaccination, smallpox, 58
Vaccine, calf lymph, 58
    cowpox, 58
    pertussis, 147
    yellow fever, 138
Vaccinia, 54
Vapors, mephitic, 43
Variola, 21, 46, 54
Vector, 97, 124, 128, 139, 151
    arthropod, 145
    insect, 47
Venereal diseases, 21, 46, 147, 155
Venice, Italy, quarantine regulations, 1374, 25
Virus, cultivation, 89
    diseases, 89
    influenza, 138
    variola, 138
Viruses, 140
    Coxsackie, 139
    filtrable, 38, 75, 88, 139
Virginia, 11, 19, 29, 81
    yellow fever in, 29
Vision, defective, 80, 83
Vital statistics, 79, 108, 130
    American pioneers in, 79, 80
Voluntary health organizations, 153, 154

W

War, Civil, 59, 70
    Revolutionary, 17
    Spanish American, 83, 86, 150
    World, I, 80, 87, 114, 127
    World, II, 127, 139, 144, 148
Warfare, biological, 160
Warres, 11
Warriors, Indian, 11
Wassermann test, 75
Water, 41
    analysis, sanitary, 119
    drinking, 95, 107
    pollution of, 69, 93, 95
    standards, bacteriological, 92
    supply, 61, 62
Waterbury, Connecticut, 16
Weather Bureau, 79
West Indies, 25, 34, 36, 48
West Virginia, 81
Wethersfield, Connecticut, 26
Whooping cough, 70, 147

Widal test, 75, 89
Wisconsin, 82
World Center for Influenza, 149
World Health Organization, 149
World War I, 80, 87, 114, 127
World War II, 127, 139, 144, 148
Wrath of God, 15, 16, 33

X

X factor in epidemiology, 49, 50
X-Ray, 75
    studies, 82

Y

Yale University, 36
Yellow fever, 12, 17, 28, 29, 30, 31,
        32, 33, 34, 35, 36, 37, 39,
        40, 41, 42, 44, 45, 47, 52,
        53, 54, 55, 56, 57, 58, 63,
        84, 88, 90, 97, 98, 99, 103,

Yellow fever—Cont'd
        104, 105, 106, 108, 138,
        143, 145, 150, 151
    conditions for continued ex-
        istence of, 104
    control, 138
    endemic, focus of, 105
    epidemic of 1793, 32
    epidemics of, 98
    influence on epidemiological
        thinking, 31
    in New York, 1668, 12
    in Philadelphia, 17, 37
    jungle, 138, 145
    role of mosquitoes in, 104
    The American Pedagogue, 28
    transmission of, 90
    vaccine, 138
Yellow Fever Commission, U. S.
    Army, 84, 106